HOME WORKOUT FOR SENIORS OVER 50+

Easy, Safe, and Fun Exercises for Lifelong Well-being

Louis Whitlock

COPYRIGHT

© **2024 by Louis Whitlock.** All rights reserved.

DISCLAIMER

The content in "Home Workout for Seniors Over 50+: Easy, Safe, and Fun Exercises for Lifelong Well-Being" is meant solely for educational and informational reasons and should not be used as a substitute for professional medical advice, diagnosis, or treatment. Always consult your physician or other trained health practitioners if you have any queries about a medical condition or before starting any exercise regimen.

The exercises and routines detailed in this book are intended for healthy adults over the age of 50. If you have any pre-existing medical illnesses, injuries, or drugs that may impair your ability to exercise, you should contact your doctor before beginning this or any other fitness program.

The author and publisher of this book accept no responsibility for any injuries or health concerns that may come from following the workout regimens and instructions described herein. By participating in the activities described in this book, you agree to do so at your own risk and accept full responsibility for any resulting injuries.

Always proceed with caution, begin gently, and make adjustments as needed to guarantee your safety and comfort. Listen to your body, and discontinue any workout that produces pain or discomfort. Your health and well-being are most important, so please prioritize safety and seek expert help when necessary.

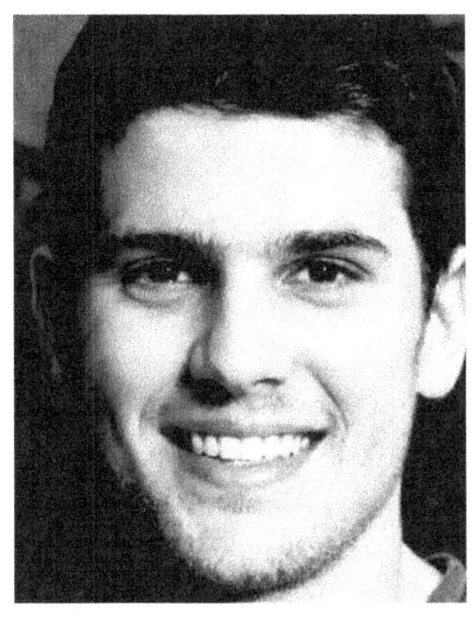

About the Author

Louis Whitlock is a very great fitness trainer with more than 20 years of expertise in the health and wellness business. His commitment to assisting people in achieving their fitness objectives has earned him a loyal and valued following

Louis Whitlock is a very great fitness trainer with more than 20 years of expertise in the health and wellness business. His commitment to assisting people in achieving their fitness objectives has earned him a loyal and valued following

Louis' fitness path began with his own transforming experience, which sparked a lifelong dedication to physical health and well-being. He holds multiple certifications in personal training, senior fitness, yoga, and functional movement. His knowledge and compassionate attitude have inspired countless elders to adopt an active lifestyle, regardless of their starting place.

TABLE OF CONTENTS

INTRODUCTION 6

Chapter 1: Essential equipment and safety considerations 9

Affordable and Space-Saving Workout Equipment 10

Tips for Safe Exercise at Home 18

How to Create a Safe Workout Space 20

Common Injuries and How to Prevent them 22

Chapter 2: Warming Up and Getting Started 24

The Importance Of Warming Up Before Exercise 25

Simple warm-up routines 27

Guidelines for starting a workout program 31

How to Monitor Progress and Adjust Routines 33

Chapter 3: Stretching for Flexibility 36

Advantages of Stretching for Seniors 37

Basic Stretching Exercises for Seniors 40

Planning a Daily Stretching Routine 46

Tips to Avoid Overstretching 50

Chapter 4: Yoga for Strength and Balance 54

An Introduction to Yoga 55

Getting Started With Yoga 58

Basic Yoga Pose and Modifications 59

Breathing exercises and relaxation 66

Breathing Techniques 66

Suggestions for Effective Breathing and Relaxation 73

Tips for Doing Yoga Safely 74

Chapter 5: Cardio Exercises for Heart Health 75

The Importance of Cardiovascular Exercise for Seniors 76

Cardiovascular Exercises for Seniors 79

Low-Impact Cardio Workouts for Seniors 81

How to gently increase cardio intensity? 87

Monitoring Heart Rate and Exercise Levels 90

INTRODUCTION

Welcome to the "Home Workout for Seniors Over 50+: Easy, Safe, and Fun Exercises for Lifelong Well-being." Whether you want to maintain your current fitness level, restore lost strength and mobility, or simply begin a new journey toward a healthier lifestyle, this book will help you every step of the way.

As we become older, staying active becomes more vital for our physical, mental, and emotional health. Regular exercise helps to preserve muscular mass, improve balance and flexibility, promote cardiovascular health, and improve general quality of life. Furthermore, it can be an effective technique for controlling chronic diseases, lowering stress, and encouraging a good attitude about life.

This book is designed exclusively for seniors over 50, focusing on safe, simple, and pleasurable workouts that may be done at home. You don't need a gym membership or pricey equipment to keep active and healthy—just a little room, some basic equipment, and a dedication to your well-being.

How To Use This Book:

Each chapter in this book focuses on a different facet of a well-rounded fitness regimen, from choosing low-cost home gym equipment to incorporating several types of exercise such as stretching, yoga, and cardio.

Begin by familiarizing yourself with the fundamental principles in Chapter 1, which covers necessary equipment and safety precautions. From there, work your way through each chapter, creating a thorough and balanced training regimen that meets your specific needs and fitness goals.

Setting Realistic Fitness Goals.

It is critical to develop attainable and realistic goals. This not only motivates you, but also allows you to track your progress. Remember that it's never too late to begin exercising, and each small step you take puts you closer to a better, more active lifestyle.

Support and Motivation

Maintaining a consistent fitness program can be difficult, especially if you are doing it alone. Consider finding a workout buddy, joining an online fitness network, or enlisting the support of family and friends to help you stay motivated and accountable. Celebrate your success, no matter how tiny, and be gentle with yourself on days when things don't go as expected.

Let us get started on this journey together. Here's to your health, happiness, and long-term well-being!

CHAPTER 1

ESSENTIAL EQUIPMENT AND SAFETY CONSIDERATIONS

AFORDABLE AND SPACE-SAVING WORKOUT EQUIPMENT

Creating an effective home gym environment does not necessitate a huge investment or a separate room. With a few inexpensive and space-saving pieces of equipment, you can undertake a variety of workouts to stay fit and healthy. Here are a few of the top choices:

1. RESISTANCE BANDS

Resistance bands are adaptable, portable, and affordable. They come in a variety of resistance levels, allowing you to progressively raise the intensity of your workouts as your strength improves.

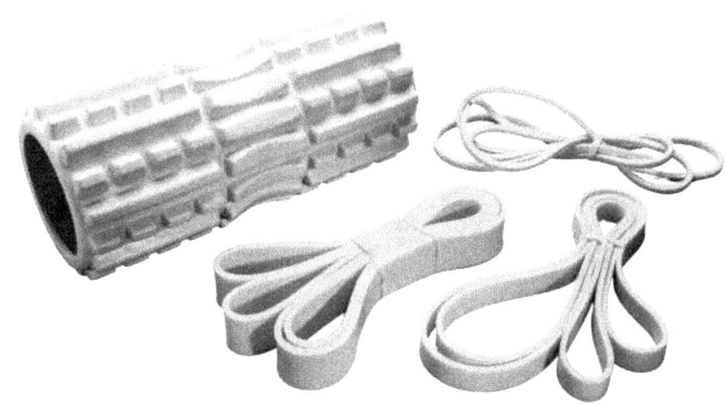

Benefits:

• Portable and lightweight
• Suitable for various muscle-targeting exercises.
• Suitable for every fitness level.

Usage Tip:

• Anchor to a door or stable object for varied activities.
• Incorporate into stretching practices for additional resistance.
• Combine several bands to boost resistance.

2. DUMBBELLS

Dumbbells are essential to any training plan. They come in a variety of weights, and adjustable dumbbells can save both space and money.

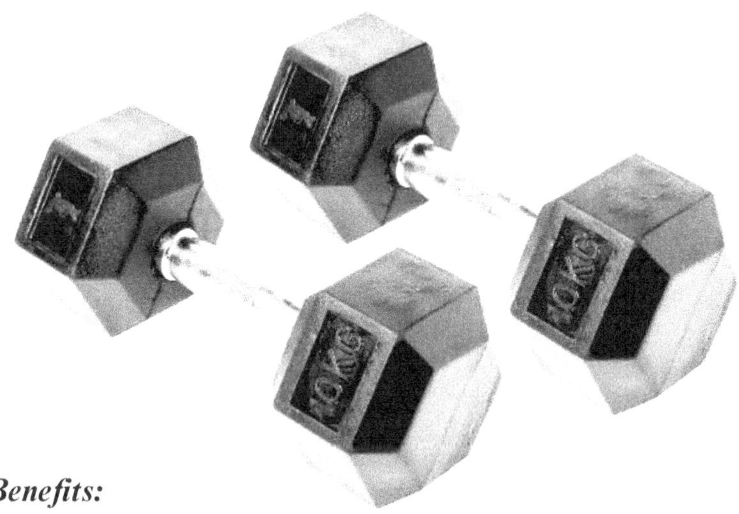

Benefits:

• Ideal for strength training
• Adaptable to various workouts
• Adjustable choices are space efficient.

Usage Tip:

• Begin with lesser weights, gradually increasing as you gain strength.
• Perform workouts such as bicep curls, shoulder presses, and weighted squats.
• Maintain appropriate form to avoid injuries.

3. EXERCISE MAT

An exercise mat creates a comfortable and safe surface for floor workouts, stretching, and yoga.

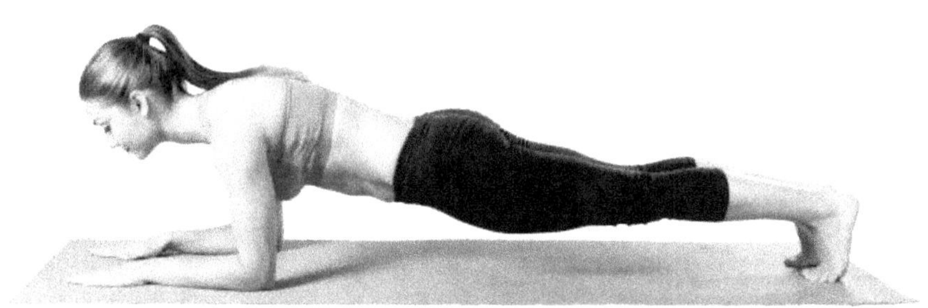

Benefits:

• Protects joints during floor exercises
• Simple to roll up and store
•Non-slip surface ensures safety

Usage Tips:

• Choose a thick mat for comfort.
• Clean periodically to preserve hygiene.
• Suitable for yoga, Pilates, and bodyweight workouts.

4. STABILITY BALL

A stability ball, often known as a Swiss ball, is ideal for core exercises and increasing balance.

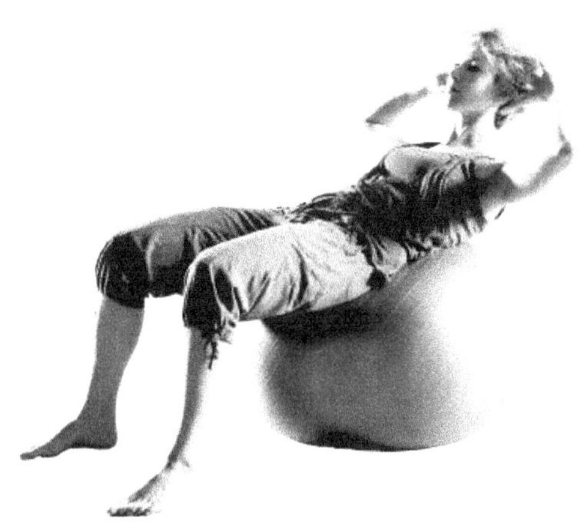

Benefits:

- Improves core strength and stability
- Suitable for various exercises.
- Functions as a chair for ergonomic seating.

Usage Tip:

- Inflate the ball properly
- Use for exercises such as ball crunches, wall squats, and seated leg lifts.
- Begin with basic exercises to adjust to the balancing needs.

5. ANKLE WEIGHTS

Ankle weights give resistance to lower-body movements, increasing their difficulty and effectiveness.

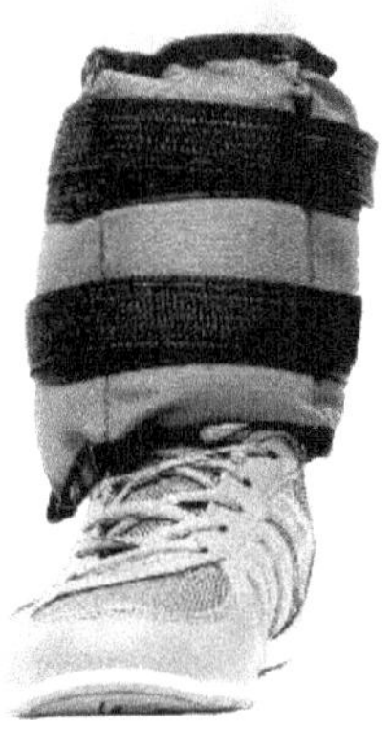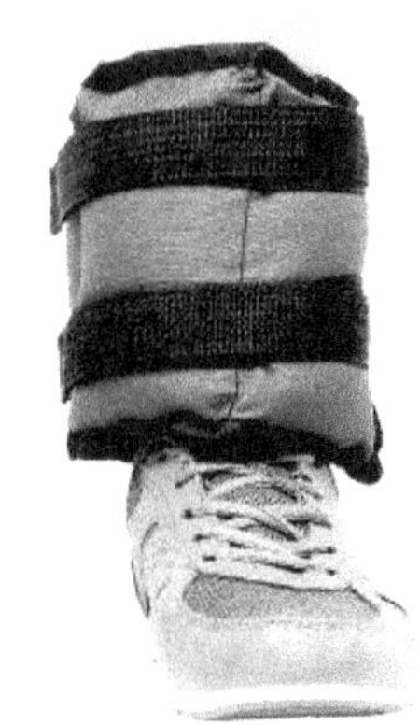

Benefits:

- Convenient storage
- Enhances leg training intensity
- Suitable for varied exercises.

Usage Tip:

- Begin with lighter weights to reduce strain.
- Use for leg lifts, walking, and other lower body exercises.
- Gradually increase weight as strength improves.

6. JUMP ROPE

Jumping rope is a terrific aerobic workout that takes very little room and equipment.

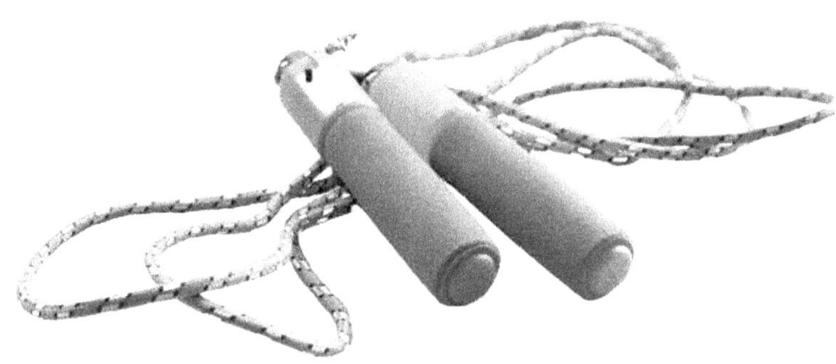

Benefits:

- Excellent for cardio fitness
- Portable and inexpensive.
- Enhances coordination and agility.

Usage Tips:

- Choose the right rope length for your height
- Begin with short sessions and progressively increase duration
- Wear appropriate footwear to protect your joints.

7. FOAM ROLLER

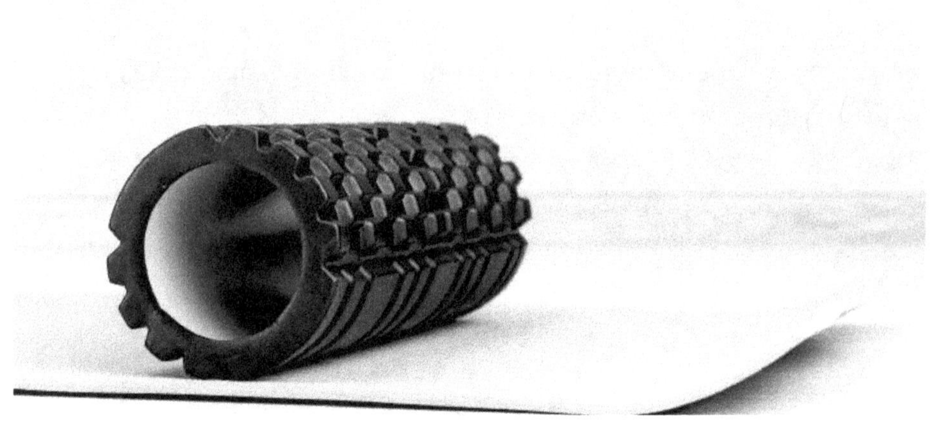

A foam roller is used for self-myofascial release, which helps to relieve muscular stiffness and increase flexibility.

Benefits:

* Promotes muscular recovery.
* Enhances flexibility and range of motion
* Compact and convenient to store

Usage Tip:

* Massage painful muscles after your workout.
* Slowly roll over tight places, pausing at vulnerable parts.
* Add to your warm-up or cool-down routine.

By combining these low-cost and space-saving pieces of equipment into your home training regimen, you may enjoy a thorough and effective fitness program without requiring a huge investment or dedicated space. Begin with a few important things, then gradually expand your collection based on your fitness objectives and tastes.

TIIPS FOR SAFE EXERCISE AT HOME

When exercising at home, it is critical to consider safety to avoid accidents and guarantee that your routines are productive. First, ensure that your training environment is safe by removing any clutter such as furniture or toys that you may trip over. Use a non-slip mat or rug to assist you stay steady, especially during balance exercises, and keep the space well-lit to avoid mishaps.

Wearing appropriate footwear and attire is also essential. Choose supportive, well-fitting shoes to protect your feet and prevent slippage, and dress in comfortable, breathable clothing that allows you to move freely. Begin your workout with a modest warm-up to prepare your body and limit the danger of injury. Gradually raise the intensity of your workouts as you gain strength, rather than pushing too hard at the start.

Proper form is essential for avoiding injuries. Learn the proper technique for each exercise by watching videos or seeking advice from a trainer if needed, and do exercises slowly and carefully to preserve control and reduce strain. Always listen to your body—if you experience intense pain or discomfort, stop exercising right away and relax, and allow your body time to recover between exercises to avoid overuse problems.

It's also crucial to stay hydrated and fuel your body correctly. Drink water before, during, and after your workout to stay hydrated, and eat a healthy diet to fuel your workouts and aid in recovery. Finally, understand your limitations and choose activities that are appropriate for your fitness level, rather than pushing yourself too hard. If you have any limitations or concerns, modify the exercises to guarantee your safety.

By following these easy safety guidelines, you may develop a safe and effective home fitness regimen that will keep you fit and healthy.

HOW TO CREATE A SAFE WORKOUT SPACE

Creating a safe training environment at home is critical for avoiding injuries and making your exercise regimen pleasurable and efficient. Here's how to create a safe workout area:

Begin by selecting a location with adequate area to move freely. Remove any debris from the area, including furniture, toys, and cords that you could trip over. Ensure that the floor is clean and clear of any slippery substances.

Next, ensure that the surface you will be exercising on is appropriate. If you're doing out on a hard floor, use an exercise mat to cushion and support your joints while lessening the impact. A non-slip mat can also help you avoid sliding while exercising.

Good lighting is vital for a safe workout environment. Make sure the location is well-lit to prevent mishaps. Natural light is preferable, but if that is not possible, utilize strong, artificial lighting.

Ventilation is another key consideration. A well-ventilated area keeps the air fresh and helps to maintain your body temperature while exercising. If possible, consider a room with open windows or use fans to circulate air.

Organize your equipment neatly. Weights, resistance bands, and other gear should be stored in a specific place to avoid tripping hazards. Using storage containers or shelves can help keep everything organized and accessible.

Finally, make sure you have a solid and safe environment to workout in. If you're doing balance exercises with a chair or stretching against a wall, make sure it's sturdy and won't move unexpectedly. Double-check that any equipment you use is in good working order and safe to use.

By following these steps, you may establish a safe and productive training room at home, allowing you to exercise with confidence and comfort.

COMMON INJURIES AND HOW TO PREVENT THEM

1. Strains and Sprains: Strains occur when muscles or tendons are overstretched or torn, whereas sprains cause ligament damage. To avoid these injuries, begin with a complete warm-up for your muscles and ligaments. Use suitable exercising routines to avoid jarring movements. To avoid overstressing your muscles, gradually raise the intensity of your workout.

2. Joint Pain: Overuse, poor technique, or inadequate support are common causes of joint pain. To avoid joint pain, choose low-impact exercises like swimming or cycling, which are softer on your joints. To prevent joint stress, choose appropriate footwear that provides good support and cushioning, and exercise with proper form.

3. Muscle soreness: Muscle soreness, also known as delayed onset muscle soreness (DOMS), can develop after beginning a new workout or increasing intensity. To avoid muscle pain, start with mild intensity and gradually increase it to allow your muscles to adjust. Stretching after exercise helps to prevent stiffness and increase flexibility. Make sure you get enough rest in between sessions to help your muscles heal.

4. Tendonitis: Tendonitis is inflammation of a tendon that is typically caused by repetitive strain or overuse. To avoid tendonitis, avoid repetitive movements or activities. Vary your workout program to rest different tendons, and utilize good technique. Do not push through pain, as this can aggravate the disease.

5. Back Pain: Back pain might be caused by bad posture, inappropriate lifting practices, or muscular imbalances. Strengthen your core muscles to help support your spine and improve posture. Proper lifting techniques include bending your knees and maintaining your back straight. Incorporate back and core workouts to improve flexibility and strength.

6. Blisters and calluses: Blisters and calluses are commonly caused by friction and pressure from ill-fitting shoes or equipment. Wear well-fitting, supportive shoes to reduce friction. If required, wear cushioned socks or protective clothing, and gradually increase the intensity and duration of your workouts so that your skin can adjust.

7. Fall and Trips: Clutter or uneven flooring in your training environment might lead to falls and trips. Keep your workout area clean and clear of impediments. Make sure the floor is even and use a non-slip mat. Be cautious of your movements and avoid exercises that may cause you to lose balance.

Understanding these common injuries and implementing these preventive measures will help you lower your risk and maintain a safe, productive training program. Always listen to your body and seek medical attention if you are experiencing chronic pain or discomfort.

CHAPTER 2
Warming Up and Getting Started

THE IMPORTANT OF WARMING UP AND EXERCISE

Warming up before exercise is an important stage in preparing your body for physical activity and avoiding injury. Here's why warming up is important:

1. Increases blood flow to the muscles: Warming up gradually raises your heart rate and improves blood supply to your muscles. This helps to give more oxygen and nutrients to your muscles, improving their function and lowering the chance of strains or injuries.

2. Increases flexibility and range of motion: A regular warm-up improves the flexibility of your muscles and tendons. This increases your flexibility and range of motion, making it simpler to do activities with proper form and lowering the risk of strains or joint injuries.

3. Prepares the Cardiovascular System: Warming up allows your cardiovascular system to adapt to the increasing demands of exercise. It gradually boosts your heart rate and helps your body adapt to the stress of physical activity, preventing unexpected spikes in heart rate and lowering your risk of cardiovascular problems.

4. Improves Mental Preparedness: A warm-up program allows you to psychologically prepare for your workout. It helps you focus on your exercise goals, improves your concentration, and fosters a positive mindset, all of which can increase your performance and motivation.

5. Decreases Muscle Stiffness: Warming up helps to alleviate muscle stiffness by raising the temperature of your muscles and enhancing their flexibility. This makes your muscles more elastic and less vulnerable to ailments such as strains and pulls.

6. Activate Key Muscle Groups: A proper warm-up focuses on the essential muscle groups you'll use during your workout. This ensures that these muscles are ready to work and helps to avoid overuse or strain during exercise.

7. Helps Prevent Injury: Warming up helps to prepare your body for more intensive action, lowering your chance of sprains, strains, and joint problems. It also helps to reduce stress on your muscles and joints by gradually introducing them into the activity.

How to Warm Up Effectively

To properly warm up, begin with 5 to 10 minutes of modest aerobic activity, such as brisk walking or jogging in place. Next, practice dynamic stretches or exercises that replicate the motions you'll be doing during your workout. For example, if you want to work out your lower body, warm up with leg swings, lunges, or easy squats.

A solid warm-up practice can help you exercise safely, perform better, and lower your chance of injury.

SIMPLE WARM-UP ROUTINES

An effective warm-up regimen gets your body ready for activity by gradually boosting your heart rate and relaxing your muscles. Here are some basic but effective warm-up routines you can follow:

1. March in Place: Begin by marching in place for 1–2 minutes. Raise your knees and swing your arms softly. This helps to gradually raise your heart rate and warm your legs.

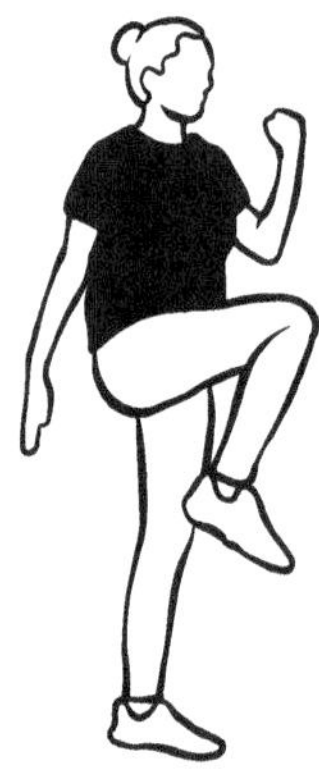

2. Arm Circles: Extend your arms to the sides and form little circles with them. Slowly raise the size of the circles. Perform 30 seconds in each direction. This workout will warm up your shoulders and arms.

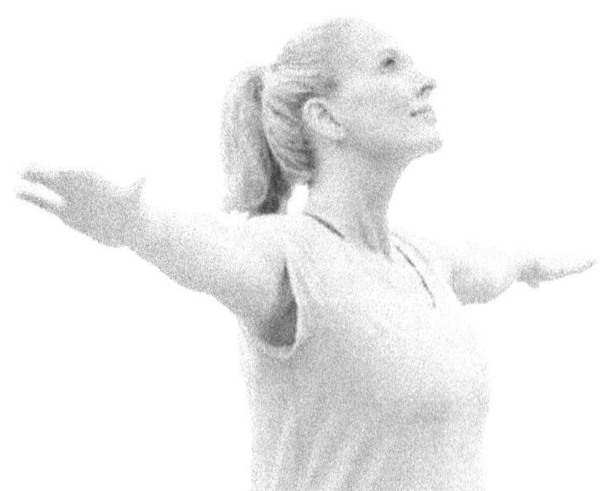

3. Leg Swings: To maintain equilibrium, hold onto a wall or a chair. Swing one leg gently forward and backward for 30 seconds before switching to the other leg. This exercise helps to loosen your hip joints and hamstrings.

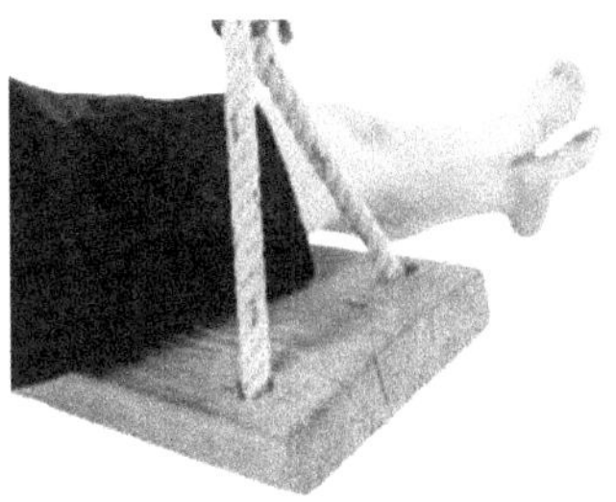

4. Gentle Side Lunges: Step to the side with one foot and bend the knee, keeping the other leg straight. Push back to the starting position and repeat on the opposite side. Perform for 1–2 minutes. This will warm up your thighs and hips.

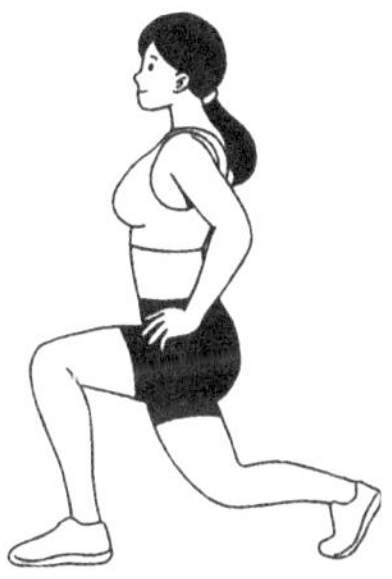

5. Torso Twists: Stand with your feet shoulder-width apart and gently twist your torso side to side. Keep your hips facing forward and allow your arms to swing naturally. Perform this for 30 seconds to warm up your core and back muscles

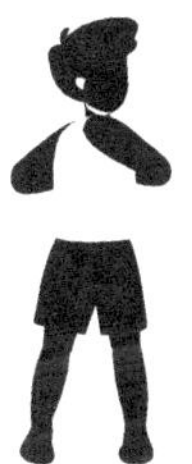

6. Heel Raises: Stand with your feet hip-width apart, slowly lifting your heels off the ground and rising to your toes. Lower back down and repeat for 1 minute. This exercise warms up your calves while improving ankle flexibility.

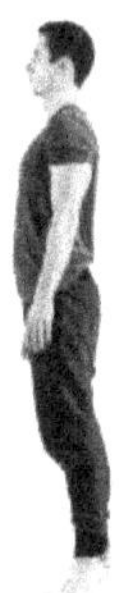

7. Gentle Jogging or Walking: If space allows, do a light jog or brisk walk for 2 to 3 minutes. This helps increase your heart rate and get your entire body ready for more intense activity.

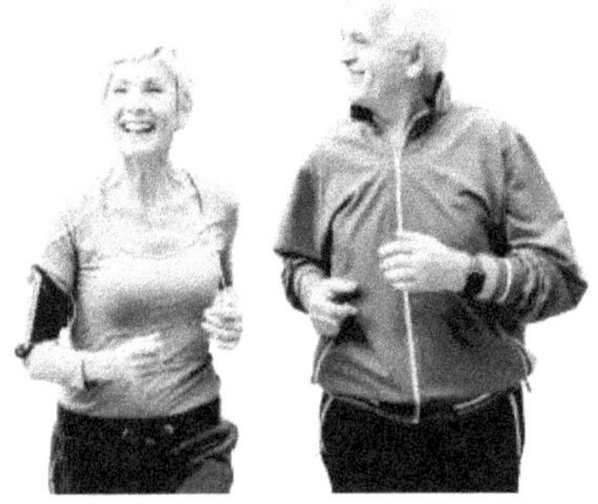

8. Shoulder Shrugs and Rolls: Lift your shoulders up towards your ears and then roll them back down in a circular motion. Do this for 30 seconds. This exercise helps relax and warm up your shoulder muscles.

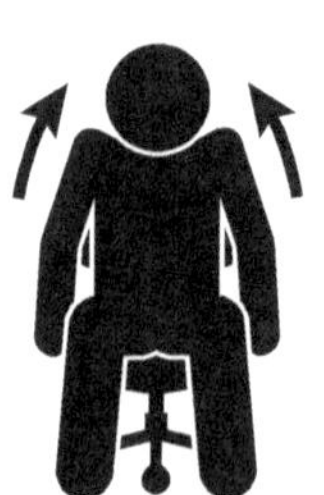

9. Hip Circles: Place your hands on your hips and make large circles with your hips, moving in both directions. Perform 30 seconds in each direction. This helps loosen your hip joints and lower back.

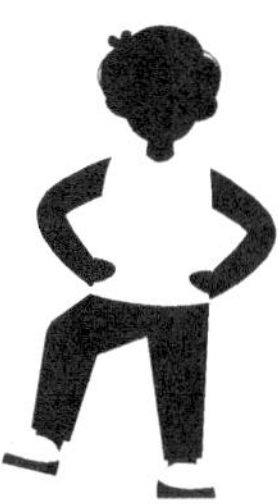

10. Dynamic Stretching: Perform dynamic stretches such as walking lunges or high knees. These stretches involve movement and help improve flexibility and range of motion. Do each stretch for 30 seconds to 1 minute.

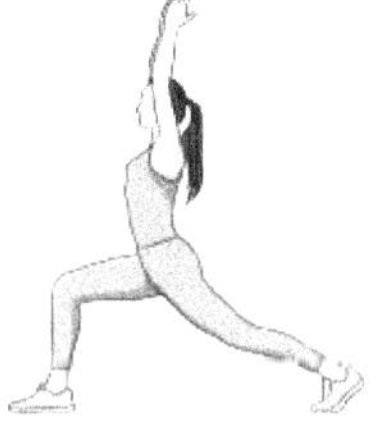

By incorporating these simple warm-up routines, you can prepare your body for exercise, enhance your performance, and reduce the risk of injury.

GUIDELINES FOR STARTING A WORKOUT SPACE

Starting a training program is a terrific approach to improve your health and well-being, especially for seniors. Here are some basic suggestions to help you get started safely and effectively:

1. Consult Your Healthcare Provider: Before beginning any new workout regimen, it's vital to talk with your healthcare professional, especially if you have any chronic diseases or concerns. They can provide recommendations on what types of exercises are safe for you and any precautions you should take.

2. Set Realistic Goals: Establish specific, achievable goals for your training routine. These might include boosting strength, increasing flexibility, or promoting general fitness. Setting realistic goals helps keep you motivated and focused.

3. Start Slowly and Gradually Increase Intensity: Begin with low-intensity workouts and progressively raise the intensity as your fitness level improves. This helps your body adjust to the new activity and minimizes the danger of damage. Start with shorter workout sessions and progressively increase the duration and intensity.

4. Select Activities You Enjoy: Choose exercises that you enjoy to boost the likelihood that you will adhere to your regimen. Walking, swimming, or taking a mild yoga session can all help make your training routine more enjoyable.

5. Use a variety of exercises: Include a variety of cardiovascular, strength, flexibility, and balance exercises in your regimen. This promotes a well-rounded training regimen and addresses several facets of physical wellness.

6. Focus on Proper Technique: Learn and apply proper techniques for each exercise to minimize injury and get the most out of your workouts. If you are unsure about good form, consult with a fitness professional who can offer advice and criticism.

7. Listen to your body: Pay attention to how your body reacts to exercise. If you suffer pain, discomfort, or strange symptoms, discontinue the exercise and seek medical attention if needed. It is critical to distinguish between normal muscle discomfort and possible injury.

8. Provide a warm-up and cool-down: Always start your workout with a warm-up to prepare your muscles and joints for activity. Finish with a cool-down to allow your body to gradually return to its resting state and increase flexibility. This can also assist to avoid discomfort and stiffness.

9. Remain Hydrated and Nourished: Drink plenty of water before, during, and after exercise to stay hydrated. Maintain a balanced diet to boost your energy and general health. Proper nutrition is essential for improving your fitness level.

10. Rest and recover: Allow time for rest and healing in between workouts. Your body requires time to mend and rebuild after training, which helps to avoid overuse injuries and assures long-term success.

HOW TO MONITOR PROGRESS AND ADJUST ROUTINES

Tracking success and changing your training regimen are critical for meeting your fitness goals and keeping your exercise program effective and fun. Here's how you can accomplish it:

1. Establish clear goals and benchmarks: Set defined, quantifiable, and achievable goals for your training routine. These goals could include increasing strength, endurance, or flexibility. Create benchmarks to help you track your progress toward these goals.

2. Maintain a Workout Log: Maintain a workout notebook or journal in which you record details about each exercise session. Include details about the exercises you did, the duration, intensity, sets, repetitions, and how you felt during and after the workout. This helps to track development and find patterns over time.

3. Track Physical Changes: Keep track of physical changes such as enhanced muscle tone, weight loss, or endurance. Take measurements (e.g., waist circumference, body weight) and progress photos on a regular basis to see how things evolve. Make sure you're monitoring consistently, such as measuring at the same time of day and in similar settings.

4. Use Fitness Apps and Tools: Consider using fitness apps or wearable devices to track a variety of parameters, including steps taken, calories burnt, heart rate, and workout length. Many applications offer useful insights and can help you create objectives and track your progress over time.

5. Evaluate Performance Regularly: Assess your performance on a regular basis against the targets you've set. For example, if you want to develop your strength, try lifting weights or doing exercises with more resistance. Check your workout diary and physical changes to evaluate if you're accomplishing your goals.

6. Listen to your body: Pay attention to how your body reacts to your workouts. Take note of any symptoms of weariness, soreness, or discomfort. If you're regularly weary or in pain, it may be time to change your routine or see a doctor.

7. Adjust the intensity and duration: As you grow, you may need to increase the intensity and duration of your workouts to keep your body challenged. Gradually increase the weights, resistance, and duration of your exercises. To minimize overexertion, keep adjustments modest.

8. Incorporate Variety: Incorporating a range of activities will help you avoid plateaus and keep your regimen interesting. Experiment with novel activities, exercise sequences, and workout designs. This variety might help you stay motivated and target different muscle regions.

9. Reevaluate Goals Periodically: Reassess your goals on a regular basis and make any necessary adjustments. As you grow, you may realize that your initial goals have been met and it is time to set new ones. Adjust your workout program to correspond with your new goals.

10. Seek Professional Help: If you're not sure how to track your progress or make modifications, see a fitness professional or personal trainer. They can provide you tailored counsel, help you set realistic objectives, and create a regimen that works for you.

By analyzing your progress on a regular basis and making strategic tweaks to your routine, you can keep your training program productive and on track with your fitness goals. This method will help you stay motivated, accomplish better outcomes, and have a more rewarding exercise experience.

CHAPTER 3

Stretching for Flexibility

ADVANTAGES OF STRETCHING FOR SENIIORS

Stretching has several benefits, especially for seniors, as it improves flexibility, mobility, and overall well-being. Here's how stretching can improve your routine:

1. Improves flexibility: Regular stretching promotes and enhances flexibility, which is critical for seniors. Increased flexibility provides for a wider range of motion in joints and muscles, making everyday tasks like reaching, bending, and walking easier and more pleasant.

2. Reduces muscle stiffness: Muscles and tendons can stiffen and lose flexibility as we become older. Stretching reduces stiffness by keeping muscles and tendons stretched and supple. This reduction in muscular stiffness can relieve discomfort and enhance overall movement.

3. Improves balance and coordination: Stretching improves flexibility and muscular function, which can help with balance and coordination. This is especially significant for elders, as improved balance lowers the chance of falls and accidents, enabling greater independence and safety in daily activities.

4. Relieves pain and discomfort: Stretching can help to alleviate pain and discomfort caused by muscle tension and stiffness. Gentle stretching can help relieve muscle tightness, joint discomfort, and tension that can build up from prolonged sitting or inactivity.

5. Supports joint health: Stretching helps to keep joints healthy by increasing the circulation of synovial fluid, which lubricates them. This can reduce joint stiffness and enhance general joint health, making movements more fluid and less painful.

6. Improves circulation: Stretching exercises promote blood flow to muscles and tissues. Improved circulation helps transport oxygen and nutrients to muscles, promoting healing and lowering the chance of injury.

7. Improves posture: Regular stretching helps to extend tight muscles and improve alignment, resulting in better posture. Good posture reduces tension on the back and neck while also improving general comfort and health.

8. Reduces stress and promotes relaxation: Stretching can have a relaxing impact on both the body and mind. Stretching in your daily routine can help to reduce stress, increase relaxation, and improve general mental health.

9. Improves Physical Performance: Stretching helps seniors perform better by enhancing muscle flexibility and range of motion. This can make physical activity more fun and less strenuous for the body.

10. Supports Functional Fitness: Stretching improves functional fitness by allowing you to execute routine chores more easily. Lifting groceries, gardening, or playing with grandchildren can all be made easier with increased flexibility and reduced muscle stiffness.

Regular stretching can give substantial benefits for seniors, including improved flexibility, balance, and general quality of life.

BASIC STRETCHING EXERCISES FOR SENIORS

Basic stretching exercises can help improve flexibility, reduce stiffness, and increase overall mobility. Here are some easy stretches that are very beneficial for seniors:

1. Neck Stretch

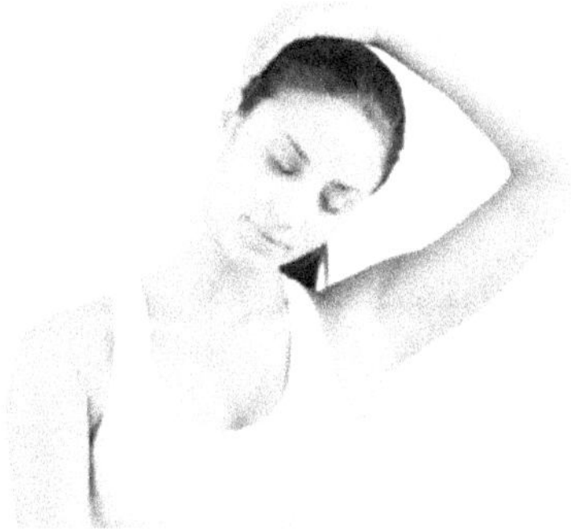

How to Do It: Sit or stand up straight. Gently tilt your head towards one shoulder, using your hand to apply light pressure as needed. Hold for 15-30 seconds, then switch to the opposite side.

Benefits: Reduces strain in the neck and shoulders.

2. Shoulder Stretch

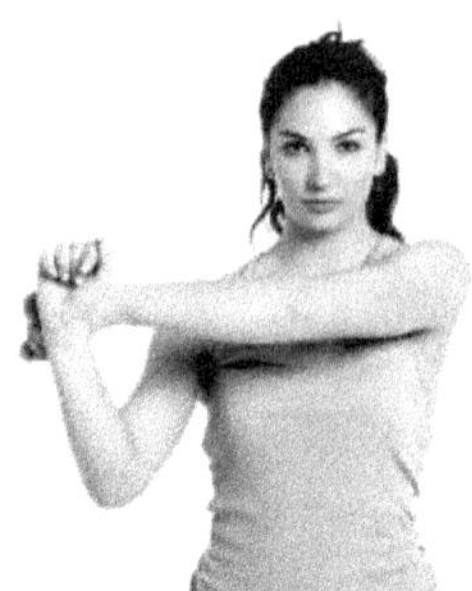

How to Do It: Place one arm across your chest and gently press the opposing arm against your body. Hold for 15-30 seconds and then switch arms.

Benefits: Stretches the shoulder muscles and increases upper body flexibility.

3. Chest Stretch

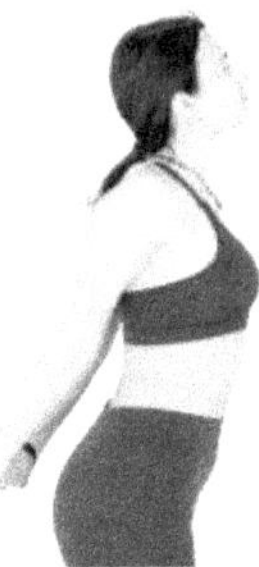

How to Do It: Position your feet shoulder-width apart. Clasp your hands behind your back and slowly raise them, opening your chest and shoulders. Hold for 15–30 seconds.

Benefits: Expands the chest and extends the front shoulder muscles.

4. Upper Back Stretch

How to Do It: Sit or stand up straight. Interlace your fingers and raise your arms in front of you, rounding your upper back. Hold for 15–30 seconds.

Benefits: Stretches the upper back and reduces tension between the shoulder blades.

5. Seated Hamstring Stretch

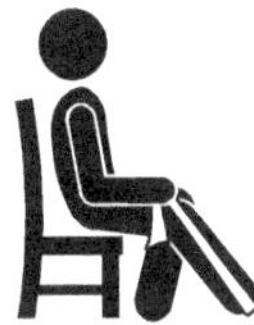

How to Do It: Sit on the edge of a chair, one leg extended straight in front of you, heel resting on the floor. Reach for your toes while maintaining your back straight. Hold for 15-30 seconds and then swap legs.

Benefits: Stretches hamstrings and lower back.

6. Calf Stretch

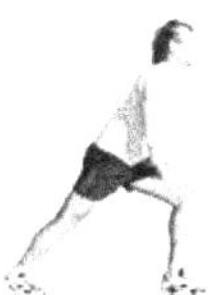

How to Do It: Stand facing a wall, one foot in front of the other. Keep your back leg straight and press your back heel down to the floor. Hold for 15-30 seconds and then swap legs.

Benefits: Stretches the calves and increases ankle flexibility.

7. Quadriceps Stretch

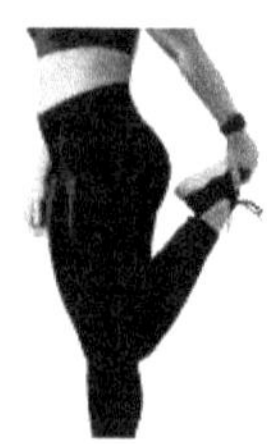

How to Do It: For added support, stand close to a chair or wall. Bend one knee and put your heel to your buttocks. Hold your ankle in your hand and slowly push your hips forward. Hold for 15-30 seconds and then swap legs.

Benefits: Stretches the front of the thigh while also improving quadriceps flexibility.

8. Side Stretch

How to Do It: Position your feet shoulder-width apart. Raise one arm overhead and slowly lean to the opposite side, feeling the stretch on your side. Hold for 15-30 seconds and then switch sides.

Benefits: Stretches the sides of the torso, increasing lateral flexibility.

9. Hip Flexor Stretch

How to Do It: Kneel on one knee and place the other foot in front, producing a 90-degree angle at both knees. Gently press your hips forwards while keeping your back straight. Hold for 15-30 seconds and then swap legs.

Benefits: Stretches the hip flexors, improving hip mobility.

10. Gentle Spine Twist

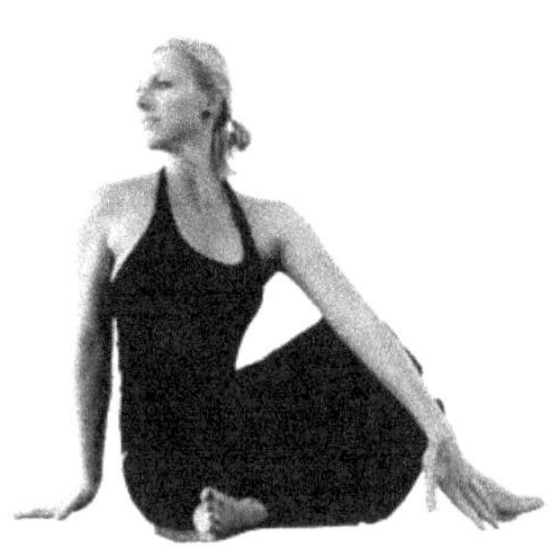

How to Do It: Sit with your back straight and legs crossed. Place one hand on the opposing leg and slowly twist your torso to that side. Hold for 15-30 seconds and then switch sides.

Benefits: Stretches the back and increases spinal flexibility.

Tips for Safe Stretching

1. Warm Up First: Begin with a light warm-up, such as walking in place, to prepare your muscles.

2. Stretch Slowly: Begin each stretch slowly and softly. Avoid bouncing or forcing your body to stretch.

3. Hold the Stretch: Hold each stretch for 15 to 30 seconds, breathing deeply and relaxing into it.

4. Listen to Your Body: Stretch until you feel mild tension rather than pain. If you experience any discomfort, relax and modify the stretch.

Incorporating these simple stretching exercises into your daily routine will help you retain flexibility, minimize muscular tension, and enhance general mobility.

PLANNING A DAILY STRECHING ROUTINE

Establishing a daily stretching regimen is a wonderful approach to improve flexibility, reduce stiffness, and promote general health. Here's a step-by-step guide to developing a stretching regimen that works into your everyday schedule:

1. Determine Your Goals: Determine what you hope to achieve with your stretching program. Goals may include increasing flexibility, lowering muscle tension, improving balance, or relieving specific discomforts. Setting defined goals allows you to adjust your program to your own needs.

2. Choose Your Stretching Exercises: Choose a range of stretches for different muscle groups. Include stretches for key areas such the neck, shoulders, back, hips, and legs. Ensure that your routine addresses all of the critical areas for balanced flexibility.

3. Set aside a specific time: Set a set time each day for your stretching routine. Whether it's in the morning to start your day, during a lunch break, or before bed, having a fixed time helps you form a habit and guarantees you don't forget to stretch.

4. Begin with a Warm-Up: Start your stretching routine with a quick warm-up to ready your muscles. Light activities like walking in place or gentle marching improve blood flow and lessen the chance of injury while stretching.

5. Incorporate a variety of stretches: Incorporate a variety of stretches to create a balanced regimen.

• **Static Stretches:** Hold each stretch for 15-30 seconds to increase flexibility.

• **Dynamic Stretches:** Use movements such as leg swings or arm circles to increase range of motion.

6. Follow a Routine Structure

Organize your routine in a logical order:

• **Warm-up:** 3–5 minutes of gentle activity.

• **Neck and Shoulder Stretches:** Begin with stretches for the upper body.

• **Back and Hip Stretches:** Transition to stretches for the back and hips.

• **Leg Stretches:** Finally, stretch your legs.

• **Cool Down:** Finish with deep breathing and mild stretching to relax.

7. Focus on Proper Technique: Stretch with proper form to avoid injury and enhance performance. Stretch slowly and softly, remaining in each posture without bouncing. Stretch until you feel mild tension rather than pain.

8. Incorporate Breathing: During each stretch, use deep, relaxed breathing to relax your muscles and increase the stretch's effectiveness. Inhale deeply before stretching, then slowly exhale while you hold the stretch.

9. Adapt the Routine as Needed: Adjust your routine to reflect your development and any changes in flexibility or physical condition. If particular stretches become easier, consider extending the length or including additional stretches into your practice.

10. Stay Consistent: Consistency is crucial to improving flexibility and overall well-being. Aim to stretch every day, even if just for a short period of time. Regular practice produces the best results over time.

11. Monitor Your Progress: Keep track of how flexible you are and how you feel after stretching. Take note of any variations in muscle tension or range of motion. Adjust your program as appropriate based on your observations and the response from your body.

Sample Daily Stretching Routine

1. Warm-up: Three minutes of marching in place.

2. Neck Stretch: 15-30 seconds per side.

3. Shoulder Stretch: Allow 15-30 seconds per arm.

4. Upper Back Stretch: 15 to 30 seconds.

5. Seated Hamstring Stretch: 15-30 seconds per leg.

6. Calf Stretch: Allow 15-30 seconds per leg.

7. Quadriceps Stretch for 15-30 seconds per leg.

8. Side Stretch: Allow 15-30 seconds per side.

9. Hip Flexor Stretch: 15-30 seconds per leg.

10. Gentle Spinal Twist: Allow 15-30 seconds per side.

11. Cool Down: Take a deep breath for one minute.

By following these instructions and adding a daily stretching regimen, you may increase your flexibility, reduce muscular tension, and feel better overall.

TIPS TO AVOID OVERSTRECHING

Overstretching can cause muscle strains, sprains, and discomfort. To stretch safely and effectively, follow these guidelines:

1. Warm up before stretching: Always start with a modest warm-up, such as strolling or gentle marching, to enhance blood flow to your muscles. Warming up prepares your body for stretching and lowers the likelihood of overstretching.

2. Stretch slowly and gradually: Begin each stretch slowly and softly. Avoid making quick or jerky motions that can strain muscles. Gradually ease into the stretch, giving your muscles time to adapt.

3. Hold stretches for the appropriate duration: Hold each stretch for 15-30 seconds, with a mild tension. Overstretching can occur when you hold stretches for too long or push yourself beyond your comfort zone.

4. Avoid Bouncing or Jerking: Avoid bouncing or jerking during stretches, a technique known as ballistic stretching. This can lead to muscle strains and injuries. Instead, utilize static stretching, which entails maintaining a stretch in a steady, controlled manner.

5. Listen to Your Body: Pay attention to how your body reacts to each stretch. You should feel minor stress or stretch, but no pain. If you feel any discomfort or sharp pain, ease out of the stretch and stop.

6. Stretch throughout your range of motion: Stretch only until you feel a moderate stretch, not to the full range of motion. Pushing too far can result in overstretching and damage. Respect your body's limitations and gradually try to increase flexibility over time.

7. Maintain proper alignment: To avoid extra strain, make sure your body is properly aligned while stretching. Keep your body in the proper position and avoid twisting or contorting it in ways that may result in overstretching.

8. Use Support When Needed: If you are having trouble attaining a stretch or keeping balance, utilize a chair, wall, or yoga block for assistance. This allows you to maintain perfect form, avoid overstretching, and still reap the benefits of the stretch.

9. Avoid stretching injured areas: If you have any injuries or stiffness, do not stretch the afflicted regions until they heal. Stretching an injured muscle or joint can worsen the situation and delay rehabilitation.

10. Gradually increase the stretch intensity: As you gain flexibility, progressively increase the intensity of your stretches. Avoid making sudden or large alterations to your daily routine. Move slowly to allow your muscles to safely adapt.

11. Include Regular Rest and Recovery: Give your muscles time to recuperate in between stretching sessions. Overstretching occurs when you strain the same muscles too frequently without enough recovery. Include rest days in your regimen to avoid overstretching and improve muscle healing.

12. Consult a professional if necessary: If you're unclear about proper stretching techniques or concerned about overstretching, talk to a fitness trainer or physical therapist. They can provide you personalized advice and help you build a safe stretching practice.

By following these guidelines, you can reduce the risk of overstretching while reaping the benefits of extending safely. Remember that moderate progress and listening to your body are essential for healthy, injury-free stretching.

CHAPTER 4

Yoga for Strength and Balance

AN INTRODUCTION TO YOGA

Yoga is an ancient discipline that blends physical postures, breathing exercises, and meditation to improve general health. Yoga, which originated in India, has spread globally as a popular form of exercise and relaxation. It is noted for emphasizing the mind-body link and providing a comprehensive approach to health and fitness.

Yoga is especially useful for elders because of its gentle and adaptive nature. It may be tailored to different fitness levels and physical ailments, making it suitable and beneficial for older persons.

The Benefits of Yoga for Senior

1. Increases flexibility: Yoga includes a number of poses that stretch and lengthen muscles, increasing general flexibility. Improved flexibility can make daily tasks like reaching and bending easier and more pleasant.

2. Improves balance and stability: Many yoga positions aim to improve balance and core strength. This can improve elders' stability, lowering the risk of falls and injury. Better balance also leads to more independence and confidence in carrying out daily chores.

3. Increases Strength: Yoga activates and strengthens multiple muscle groups through weight-bearing positions and body resistance. Regular practice can help maintain and increase muscle strength, which benefits joint health and general physical function.

4. Promotes joint health: Yoga's gentle motions and stretching can assist maintain joint flexibility and minimize stiffness. This might be especially advantageous for seniors suffering from arthritis or other joint-related disorders.

5. Enhances posture: Yoga stresses good alignment and body awareness, which can help improve posture. Better posture relieves tension on the back and neck, allowing a more comfortable sitting and standing position.

6. Lowers Stress and Increases Relaxation: Yoga involves deep breathing and relaxation techniques to reduce stress and boost mental health. These routines help boost mood, reduce anxiety, and increase calm.

7. Supports Cardiovascular Health: Regular yoga practice can boost circulation, lower blood pressure, and improve overall cardiovascular health. This easy activity promotes heart health while exerting minimal strain on the body.

8. Increases Respiratory Function: Breathing exercises, or pranayama, are an essential part of yoga. They improve lung capacity, oxygenation, and general respiratory function, resulting in healthier breathing patterns.

9. Increases Sleep Quality: Yoga can help you sleep better by reducing tension and fostering calm. Gentle stretching and breathing exercises before bedtime can help to relax the mind and prepare the body for a good night's sleep.

10. Promotes mindfulness and body awareness: Yoga promotes mindfulness and body awareness, allowing seniors to stay connected to their physical and mental states. This greater awareness can result in improved self-care and a more optimistic attitude on life.

GETTING STARTED WITH YOGA

1. Select a Class for elders: Look for yoga classes that are explicitly developed for elders or that offer modifications to accommodate different fitness levels. Many community centers and gyms offer mild yoga programs appropriate for senior persons.

2. Begin with soft Poses: Begin with simple, soft poses that promote flexibility, balance, and relaxation. Chair Pose, Cat-Cow Stretch, and Seated Forward Bend are ideal for beginners.

3. Use Props for Support: Yoga props such as chairs, blocks, and straps can offer stability and make poses more accessible. Don't be afraid to use props to maintain proper form and comfort.

4. Listen to Your Body: Practice yoga mindfully and pay attention to your body's suggestions. Avoid pushing through discomfort or pain, and adjust poses as needed.

5. Consult a Professional: If you have any health problems or conditions, speak with your doctor before beginning a yoga practice. A trained yoga instructor can also provide instruction and changes based on your specific needs.

Yoga provides various benefits for elders, including increased flexibility, balance, strength, and overall well-being. By including yoga into your routine, you can live a more active, balanced, and calm life.

BASIC YOGA POSE AND MODIFICATIONS

Yoga positions can be modified to accommodate a variety of fitness levels and physical problems. Starting with fundamental postures and making changes can help elders practice safely and effectively. Here are some basic yoga positions, with modifications to make them more accessible:

1. Mountain pose (Tadasana)

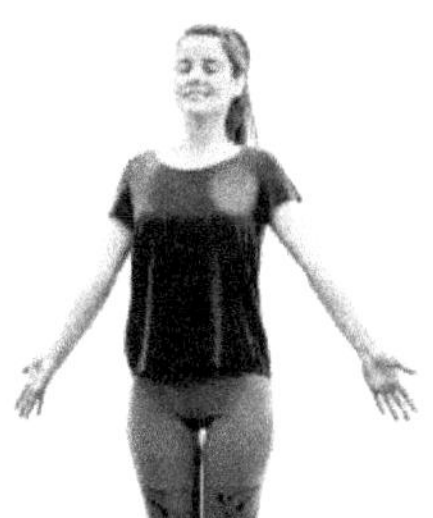

• **How to Do It:** Stand with your feet together or slightly apart and your arms by your sides. Engage your thighs, raise your chest, and stretch your spine. Keep your weight evenly spread across both feet.

• **Modification:** Use a chair or a wall for support if necessary. Concentrate on balancing your body and breathing deeply.

2. Chair pose (utkatasana)

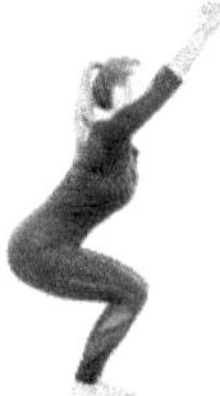

• **How to Do It:** Position your feet hip-width apart. Bend your knees as if you were sitting back in a chair, maintaining your chest up and your weight in your heels. Reach your arms overhead or keep them by your sides.

• **Modification:** Sit on the edge of a chair and elevate one leg at a time, maintaining your back straight. Use the chair to help you gain strength.

3. Cat-Cow Stretch (Marjaryasana–Bitilasana)

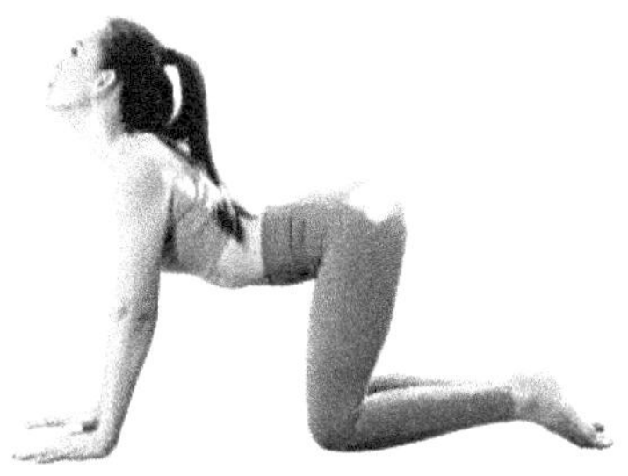

How to Do It: Beggin on your hands and knees, wrists under shoulders and knees under hips. Inhale, arch your back, and raise your head in Cow Pose. Exhale, round your spine, and tuck your chin (cat pose). Transfer between these two spots slowly.

If getting on all fours is too unpleasant, perform this stretch while sitting on a chair or using a bolster for support.

4. Seated Forward Bend (Paschimottanasana).

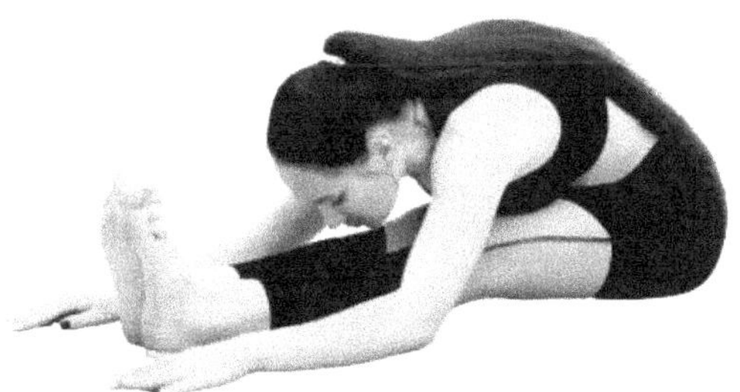

How to Do It: Sit with your legs straight in front of you. Inhale, lengthen your spine, then exhale, aiming for your toes. Maintain a straight back and prevent curving the spine.

Modification: Place a cushion or blanket on your legs and reach for it instead of your toes. This lessens the stretch tension while providing support.

5. Warrior I (virabhadrasana I)

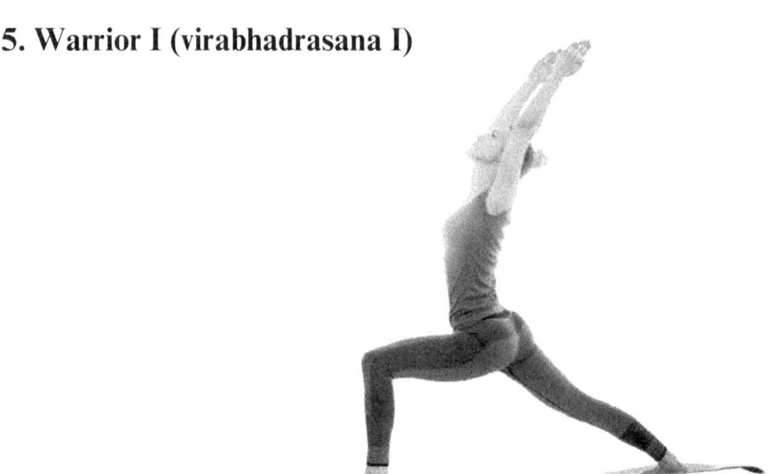

How to Do It: Take one step back, keeping the front knee bent and back leg straight. Reach your arms upwards while maintaining your shoulders relaxed. Make sure your front knee is aligned with your ankle.

If pressing down on your back heel causes discomfort, keep it raised. If necessary, balance on a chair or against a wall.

6. Warrior 2 (Virabhadrasana II)

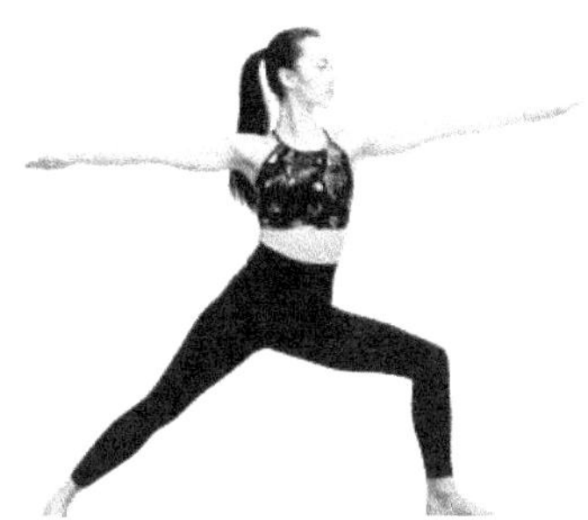

How to Do It: Start in Warrior I and open your hips and shoulders to face the side. Extend your arms parallel to the floor, palms down. Bend your front knee and keep your back leg straight.

Shorten the distance between your feet if the pose is difficult. For stability, use a chair or a wall, and pay close attention to alignment.

7. Tree pose (Vrksasana)

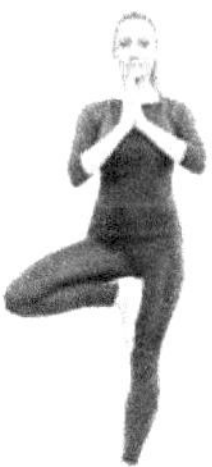

How To Do It: Stand with your feet together. Shift your weight to one foot and place the other on the inner thigh or calf. Bring your hands together at the chest or extend them overhead.

Modification: Hold this posture with your foot resting on your ankle, or use a chair for support. Hold on to a chair or a wall for balance while practicing.

8. Bridge Pose (Setu Bandhasana).

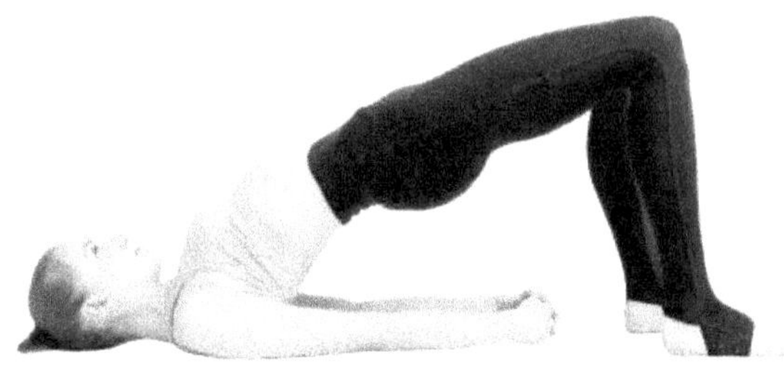

How to Do It: Lie on your back, knees bent, and feet hip width apart. Lift your hips toward the ceiling while pressing your feet onto the floor. Hold your hands behind your back or at your sides.

Modification: Place a block or pillow beneath your sacrum for support, lowering the intensity of the position. Only lift your hips as high as you can comfortably.

9. Legs Up the Wall Pose (Viparita Karani)

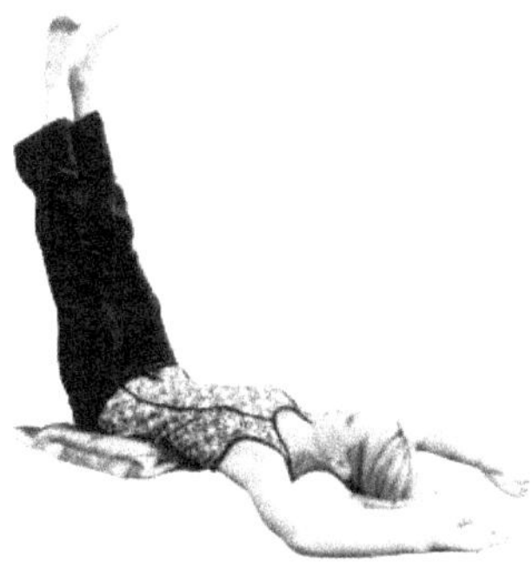

Sit close to a wall, then lie on your back with your legs swinging up the wall. Adjust your distance from the wall until you find a comfortable position. Rest your arms by your sides.

Modification: Place a folded blanket or bolster beneath your hips to provide extra support and relieve any tension.

10. Corpse Pose (Savasana).

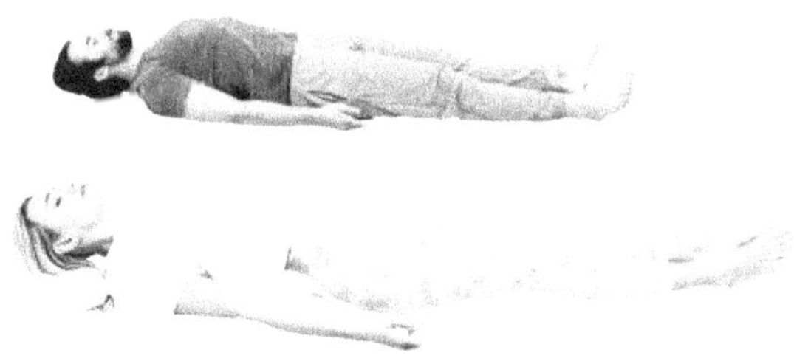

How to Do It: Lie on your back, legs extended, arms at your sides, palms up. Close your eyes and concentrate on deep, relaxing breathing. Allow your body to completely relax.

Modification: For extra comfort, place a bolster or blanket under your knees, especially if laying flat is difficult.

Tips to Practice Yoga Safely:

1. Listen to Your Body: Stretch until you feel mild tension rather than pain. Modify positions as needed to fit your comfort level.

2. Use Props: Yoga blocks, belts, chairs, and blankets can help make poses more accessible while also providing support.

3. Move Slowly: To reduce strain or injury, make slow transitions between poses.

4. Consult a Professional: If you have any health issues or conditions, speak with a healthcare provider or a skilled yoga instructor for specific advice.

By incorporating these basic postures and modifications into your practice, you may reap the benefits of yoga while keeping your routine safe and personalized to your specific needs.

BREATHING EXERCISES AND RELAXATION

Breathing methods and relaxation exercises are critical components of yoga and overall health. They promote stress management, mental clarity, and physical health. Focusing on good breathing and relaxation can help elders achieve a variety of benefits, including enhanced oxygenation, reduced anxiety, and greater sleep quality. Here's an overview of major breathing techniques and relaxation strategies appropriate for seniors:

Breathing Techniques

1. Diaphragmatic breathing (or abdominal breathing)

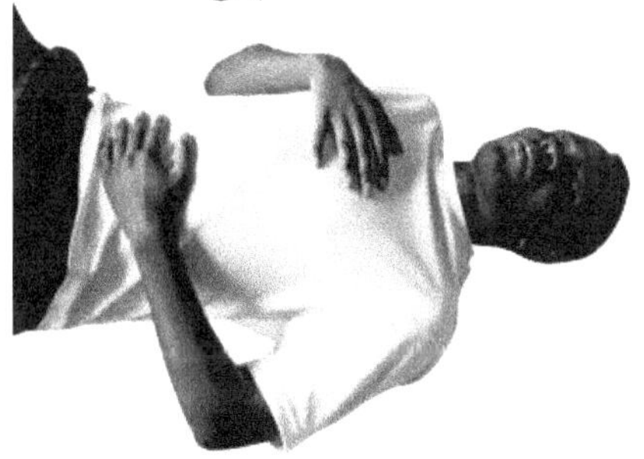

How to Do It: Sit or lie down in a comfortable position. Place one hand on your chest, the other on your abdomen. Inhale deeply through your nose, feeling your abdomen rise as your lungs fill with air. Exhale slowly through your mouth, allowing your abdomen to fall. Ensure that your chest remains reasonably still as your abdomen moves.

Benefits: Increases oxygen intake, improves relaxation, and lowers stress by activating the diaphragm.

2. Box Breath (Square Breathing)

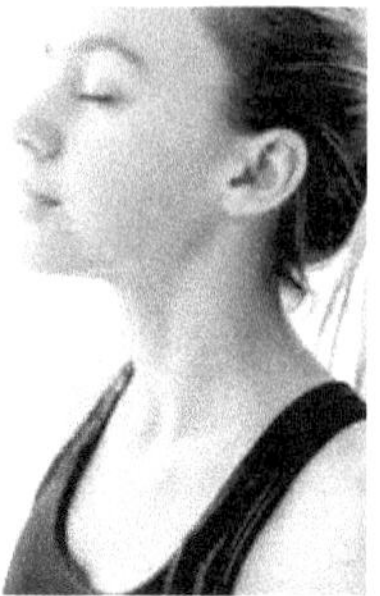

How to Do It: Take a comfortable seat or lie down. Inhale slowly through your nose for a count of four. Hold your breath for a count of four. Exhale slowly through your mouth for a count of four. Pause and hold your breath for another four counts before repeating the cycle.

Benefits: Relaxes the mind, enhances concentrate, and regulates breathing patterns. It helps to manage anxiety and tension.

3. 4-7-8 Breathing

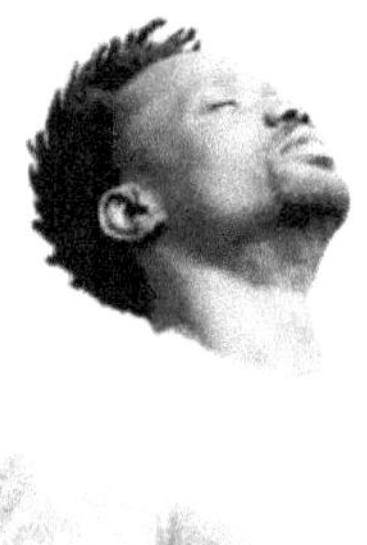

How to Do It: Sit or lie down in a comfortable position. Inhale gently through your nose for a count of four. Hold your breath for a count of seven. Exhale completely through your mouth for a count of 8. Repeat the cycle for a few minutes.

Benefits: Increases relaxation, improves sleep, and lowers stress by extending the exhale phase, which activates the parasympathetic nervous system.

4. Alternate Nostril Breathing (Nadi Shodhana)

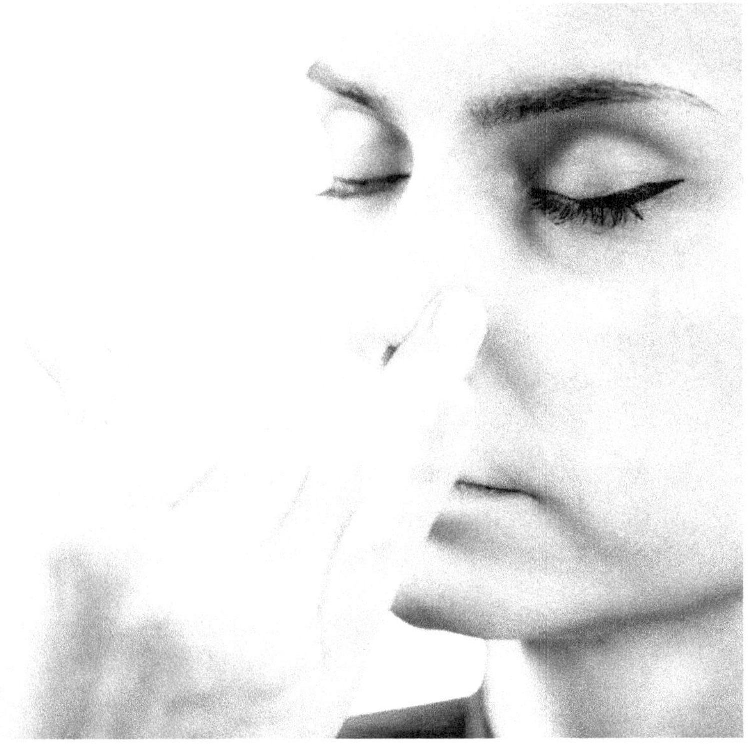

How to Do It: Sit comfortably, with your spine straight. Use your right thumb to seal your right nostril. Inhale deeply from the left nostril. Close your left nostril with your right ring finger, then release it. Exhale from your right nostril. Inhale via your right nose, then switch to exhaling through your left nostril. Continue this pattern.

Benefits: Stabilizes the neurological system, soothes the mind, and enhances respiratory function. It can also promote mental clarity and emotional stability.

Relaxation techniques

1. Progressive muscle relaxation

How to Do It: Sit or lie down in a comfortable position. Begin with your feet and work your way up the body. Tense each muscle group (feet, legs, abdomen, hands, arms, shoulders, neck, and face) for 5-10 seconds before releasing and relaxing for 20-30 seconds. Concentrate on the feeling of relaxation in each muscle group.

Benefits: Reduces physical tension, relieves stress, and raises awareness of muscular relaxation.

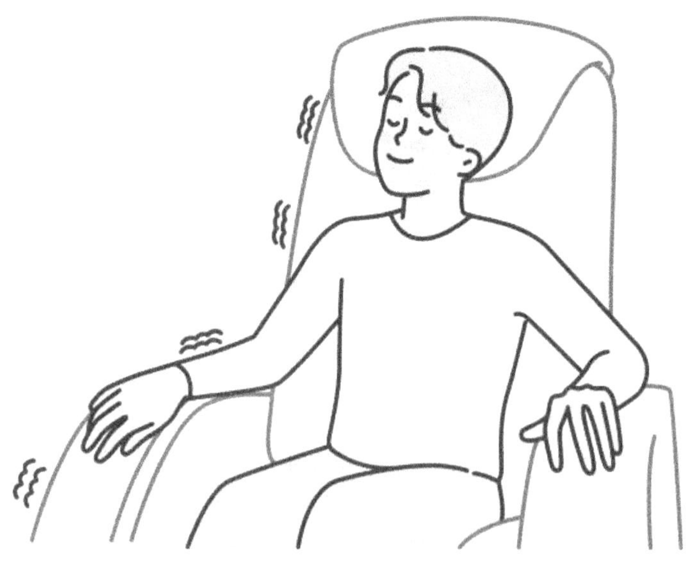

2. Guided Visualization

How to Do It: Make yourself comfortable by sitting or lying down. Close your eyes and take some deep breaths. Imagine yourself in a tranquil and pleasant environment, such as a beach or garden. Visualize the sights, sounds, and sensations of this location. Allow yourself to be in this relaxing setting for a few minutes.

Benefits: Increases relaxation, decreases tension, and increases mental clarity by engaging the imagination in a calming manner.

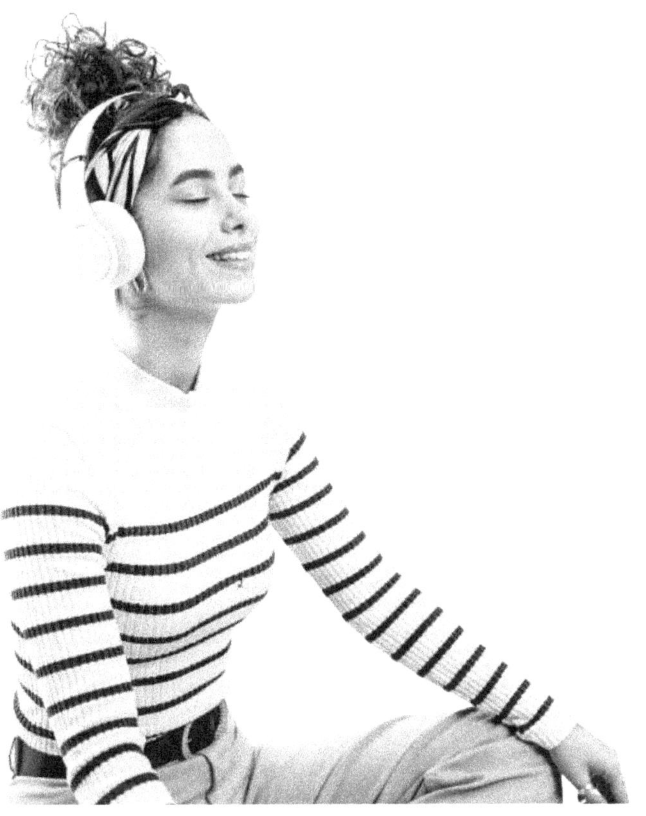

3. Body Scan Meditation

How to Do It: Take a comfortable lie-down or sitting position. Close your eyes and take some deep breaths. Bring your focus to various regions of your body, beginning with your toes and progressing to your head. Notice any sensations or tightness in any region and intentionally release them. Repeat the process until you have scanned your complete body.

Benefits: Improves body awareness, encourages relaxation, and aids in the identification and release of tension point.

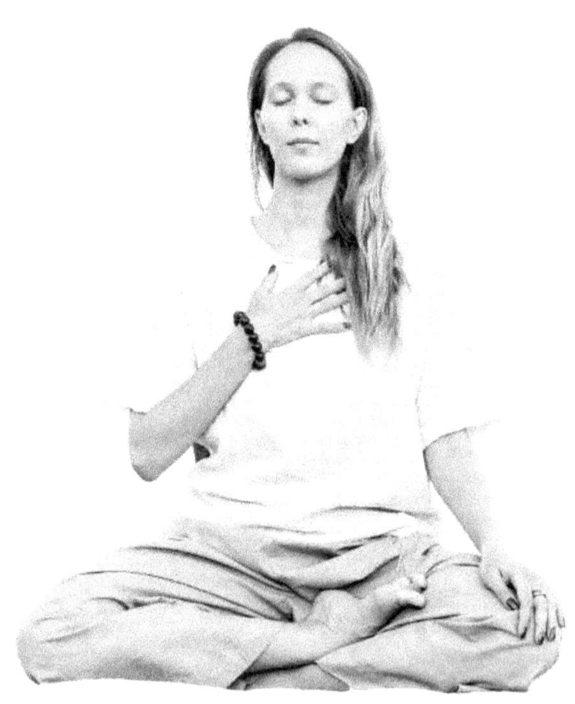

4. Mindful Meditation

How to Do It: Sit or lie down in a comfortable position, back straight. Close your eyes and concentrate on your breathing, noticing each inhalation and exhalation. If your mind wanders, softly return your attention to your breathing. Practice for a few minutes every day.

Benefits: Improves mental clarity, decreases stress, and fosters feelings of peace and presence.

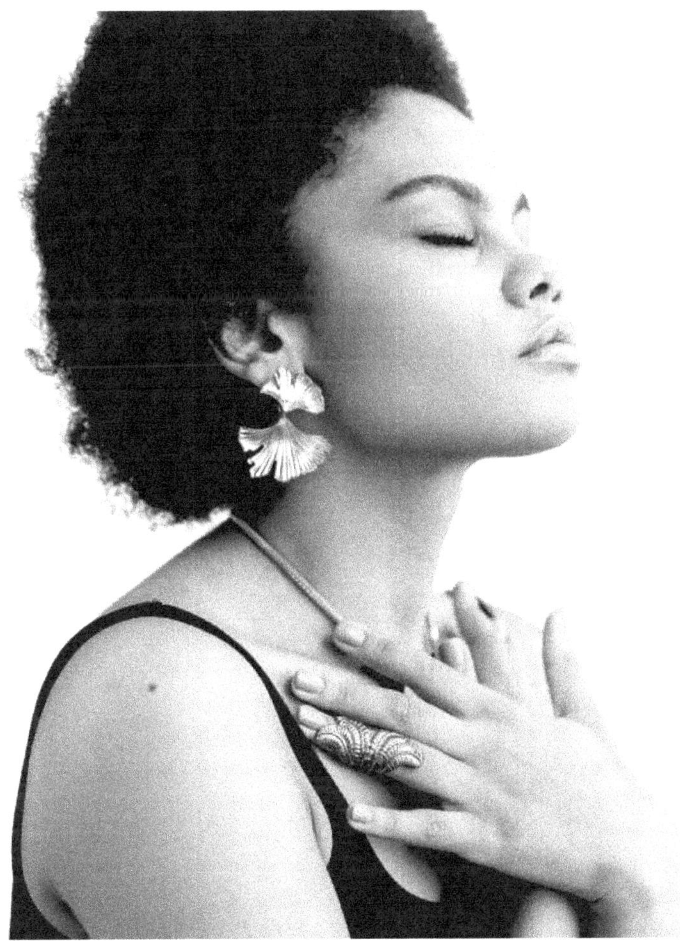

SUGGESTIONS FOR EFFECTIVE BREATHING AND RELAXTION

1. Practice Regularly: Incorporate these strategies into your everyday practice for the best results. Consistent practice promotes relaxation skills and overall well-being.

2. Find a Comfortable Position: Select a comfortable and supportive position for both breathing and relaxation exercises. Use cushions or props as needed.

3. Stay Mindful: Pay attention to your breathing and physiological sensations to stay present and improve the effectiveness of the exercises.

4. Be Patient: It may take time to reap the full benefits of these routines. Approach them with patience and an open mind.

By implementing these breathing techniques and relaxation practices into your everyday routine, you can experience increased relaxation, less stress, and better overall health.

TIPS FOR DOING YOGA SAFELY

1. Listen to Your Body: Adjust poses to your degree of comfort and avoid pushing through pain.

2. Use Props: Props like blocks, straps, and chairs can help make poses more accessible while also providing support.

3. Practice Mindfully: To make your practice more successful, focus on appropriate alignment and breath control.

4. Consult a Professional: If you have any health issues or conditions, seek advice from a certified yoga teacher.

Seniors can safely enjoy the many advantages of yoga, including better flexibility, balance, and relaxation, provided they follow these example practices and make any necessary adaptations.

CHAPTER 5

Cardio Exercises for Heart Health

THE IMPORTANCE OF CARDIOVASCULAR EXERCISE FOR SENOIRS

Cardiovascular exercise, also known as cardio, consists of activities that increase the heart rate and improve the efficiency of the cardiovascular system. Cardiovascular activity is essential for seniors to maintain their overall health and well-being. Here's why cardiovascular exercise is crucial, especially for seniors:

1. Improves Heart Health: Cardiovascular activity makes the heart muscle stronger, allowing it to pump blood more efficiently. Regular aerobic exercise lowers blood pressure and reduces the risk of heart disease by improving blood circulation and lowering cholesterol levels.

2. Boosts Circulation: Cardio exercises increase circulation throughout the body. Better circulation implies that oxygen and nutrients are transported more effectively to tissues and organs, potentially improving general physical function and energy levels.

3. Supports weight management: Regular cardiovascular activity helps to burn calories and keep a healthy weight. Weight management is critical for seniors to avoid obesity, which can lead to a variety of health conditions including diabetes and joint problems.

4. Improves lung function: Cardiovascular exercises increase lung capacity and efficiency. Improved lung function enhances oxygen intake and promotes overall respiratory health. This is especially advantageous for seniors who suffer from chronic obstructive pulmonary disease (COPD) or asthma.

5. Boosts Mental Health: Regular cardiovascular exercise has been demonstrated to boost mood and alleviate the symptoms of anxiety and sadness. The production of endorphins during exercise enhances feelings of well-being and mental clarity.

6. Improves cognitive function: Cardiovascular exercise has been related to better cognitive function and reduced risk of cognitive decline. It promotes memory, focus, and overall brain health by increasing blood flow to the brain.

7. Increases energy levels: Regular aerobic activity can increase overall vitality and lessen feelings of weariness. Seniors who improve their cardiovascular fitness may feel more energized and capable of participating in regular activities.

8. Supports joint health: Low-impact cardiovascular exercises like walking or cycling can help keep joints healthy and flexible. Exercise lubricates the joints and strengthens the muscles surrounding them, reducing stiffness and increasing mobility.

9. Enhances Sleep Quality: Regular aerobic activity can help improve sleep patterns and overall sleep quality. Better sleep promotes general health and well-being.

10. Improves Social Interaction: Group aerobic activities, such as walking clubs or fitness programs, can be socially beneficial. Social engagement and support can boost motivation and enjoyment, making exercise more appealing and sustainable.

CARDIOVASCULAR EXERCISES FOR SENIORS

1. Walking is a low-impact and easily accessible form of cardio. It can be done indoors or outside and is easily adaptable to all fitness levels.

2. Cycling: Whether on a stationary bike or a conventional bicycle, cycling is easy on the joints and gives a strong cardiovascular workout.

3. Swimming: Swimming is a full-body workout that is gentle on the joints due to the buoyancy of the water.

4. Dancing: A pleasant activity to raise the heart rate and improve coordination. Many community centers provide dance courses specifically for elders.

5. Elliptical Trainer: A low-impact machine that gives a full-body workout while minimizing joint stress.

6. Chair activities: For persons with restricted mobility, seated cardio activities can provide cardiovascular benefits while remaining safe.

Suggestions for Safe Cardiovascular Exercise

1. Begin Slowly: Start with shorter sessions and progressively increase duration and intensity as your fitness improves.

2. Warm Up and Cool Down: Use warm-up and cool-down times to avoid injury and ease into and out of your workout.

3. Stay Hydrated: Drink plenty of water before, during, and after exercise to keep yourself hydrated.

4. Wear Proper Footwear: To lower your chance of injury, wear supportive, comfortable shoes.

5. Listen to Your Body: Pay attention to how your body reacts to exercise and alter the intensity as necessary. If you have any health concerns, speak with your doctor.

Regular cardiovascular exercise can greatly improve your health, energy levels, and overall quality of life. Seniors can get the various benefits of cardio by selecting enjoyable and appropriate activities that keep them active and healthy.

LOW-IMPACT CARDIO WORKOUTS FOR SENIORS

Low-impact cardio exercises are good for seniors since they deliver cardiovascular benefits while putting less stress on joints. These activities promote heart health, increase energy, and improve general fitness without putting undue strain or danger of injury. Here are some great low-impact aerobic routines appropriate for elders.

1. Walking: Walking is a basic but effective kind of low-impact cardio. It can be done indoors on a treadmill or outside in a park or around the block.

Benefits: Improves cardiovascular health, elevates mood, and increases endurance. The tempo and duration can be easily adjusted to accommodate different fitness levels.

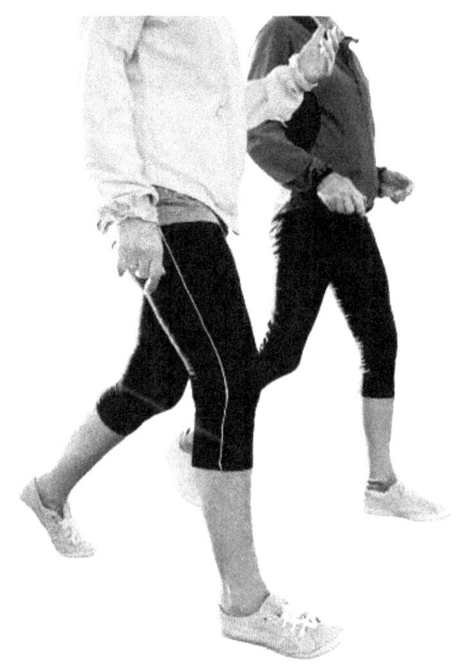

2. Cycling: Cycling can be done with either a stationary bike or a conventional bicycle. Cycling is low-impact, which decreases stress on the knees and hips.

Benefits: Improves cardiovascular fitness, strengthens lower-body muscles, and increases joint mobility. Stationary bikes frequently include changeable resistance settings, allowing for personalized workouts.

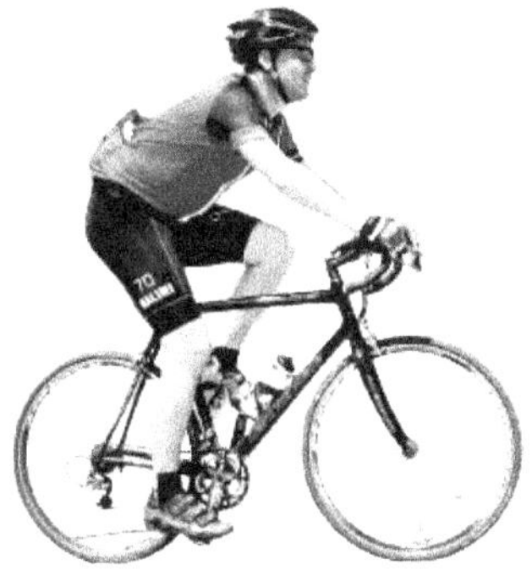

3. Swimming: Swimming is a total-body workout with little strain on the joints. It includes a variety of strokes and actions that work multiple muscle groups.

Benefits: Boosts cardiovascular endurance, strengthens muscles, and increases flexibility. The buoyancy of the water provides support for the body and lowers the risk of damage

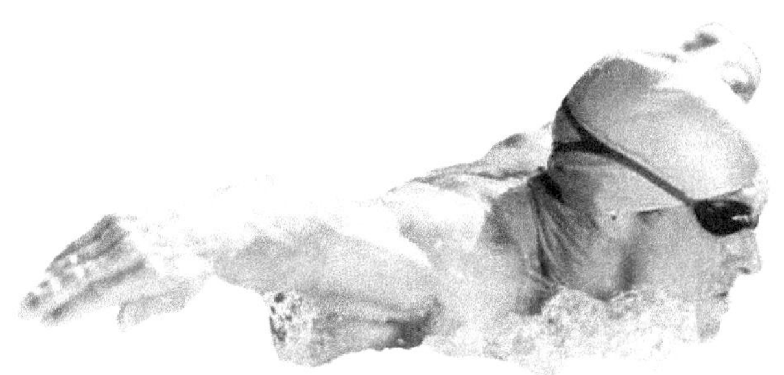

4. Water aerobics: Water aerobics are aerobic activities done in a swimming pool. It involves exercises like water jogging, jumping jacks, and arm movements.

Benefits: Provides resistance training while reducing joint tension, improving cardiovascular health, and increasing flexibility. The water's resistance aids in muscle strength development without causing excessive impact.

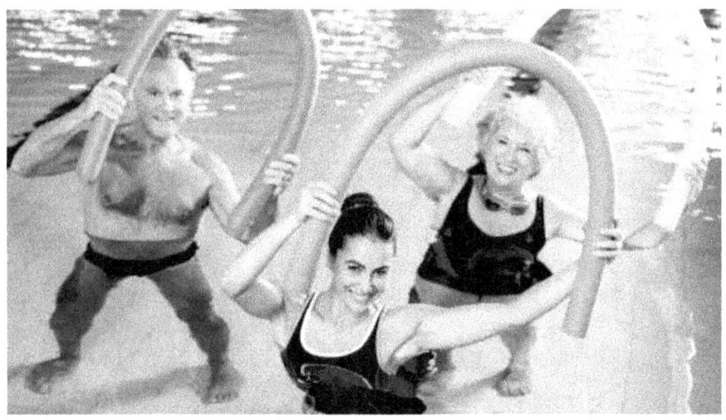

5. Elliptical Trainer: An elliptical trainer mimics walking or running with a smooth, gliding action. The foot pedals follow an elliptical route, which reduces joint impact.

Benefits: Provides a low-impact cardiovascular workout while also engaging the upper body (if the machine includes handlebars). Adjustable settings allow for different intensity levels.

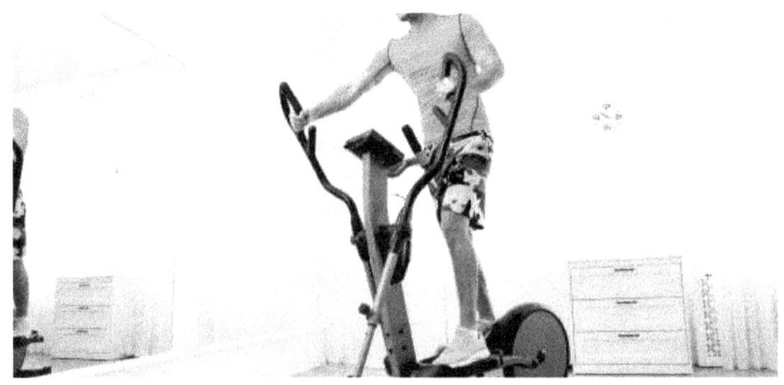

6. Chair Exercises: Chair workouts are aerobic movements done while sitting in a solid chair. Examples include seated marching, leg lifts, and seated jumping jacks.

Benefits: Helps persons with restricted mobility maintain physical activity while also providing cardiovascular advantages. Chair exercises are mild on the joints and can be tailored to specific needs.

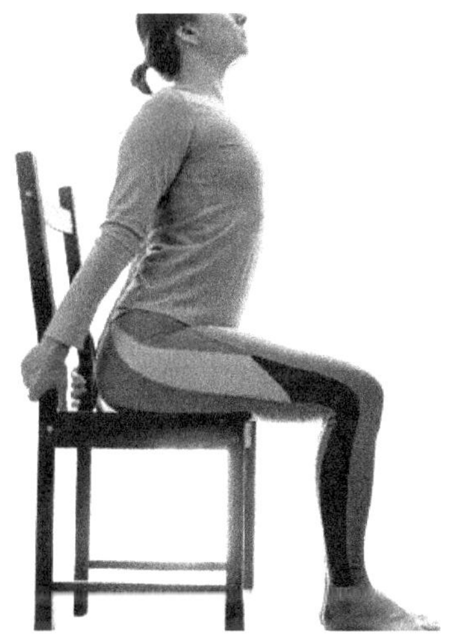

7. Low-impact Dance: Low-impact dance involves moderate routines that emphasize fluid movements and rhythm. Ballroom or line dance can be modified to lessen impact.

Benefits: Increases cardiovascular fitness, coordination, and balance. Dance routines can be changed to suit various fitness levels and interests.

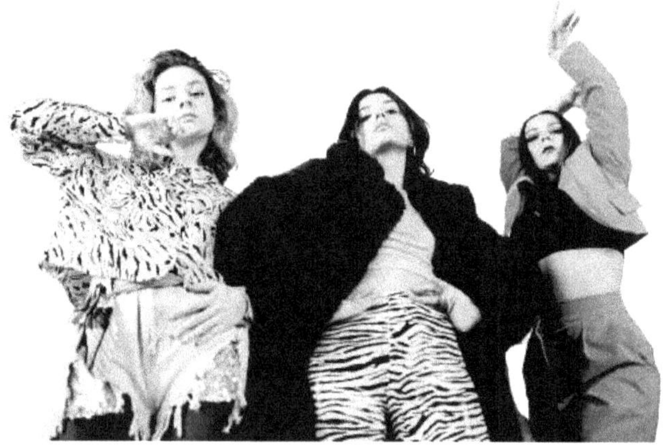

8. Step Touch: Step touch consists of stepping to the side and touching the other foot to the side. It can be done at a slow or medium pace.

Benefits: Increases cardiovascular endurance, boosts coordination, and is gentle on the joints. This exercise can be done standing or seated, as needed.

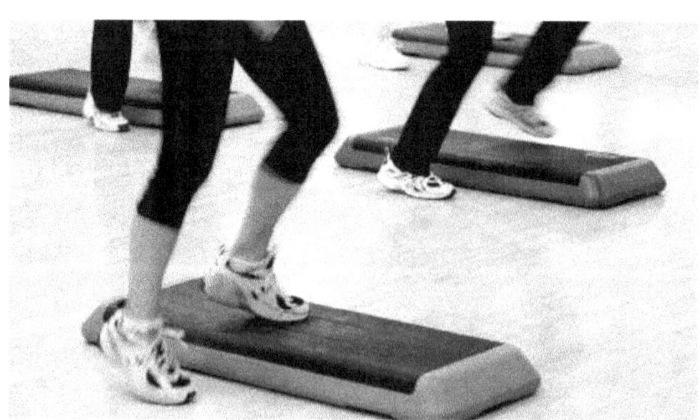

9. Gentle Hiking: Gentle hiking on level or gently sloping terrain gives a low-impact cardiovascular workout. Choose trails with even surfaces to reduce joint stress.

Benefits: Improves cardiovascular health, develops lower body muscles, and allows you to enjoy nature. Using walking poles might provide extra support.

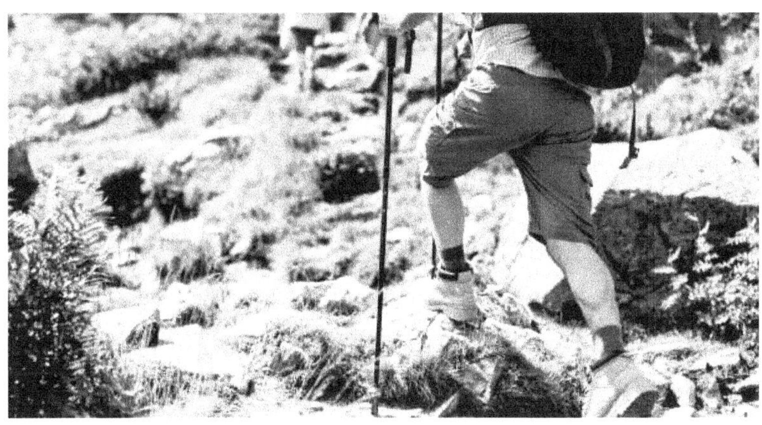

10. Tai Chi: Tai Chi is a gentle martial technique that combines slow, controlled motions with deep breathing. It is frequently done in a fluid succession.

Benefits: include better cardiovascular health, balance, flexibility, and mental relaxation. Tai Chi is ideal for elderly due to its moderate impact.

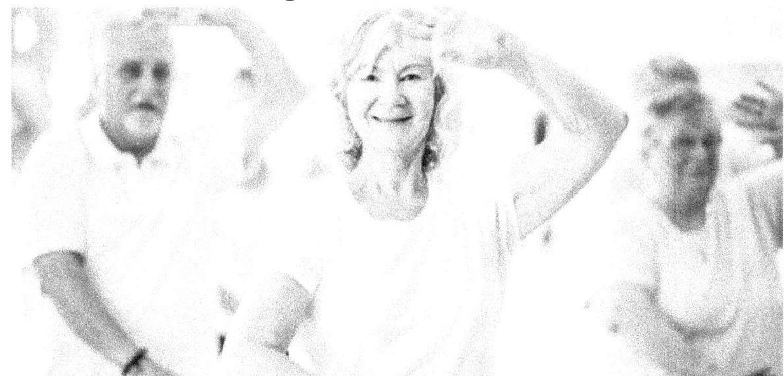

HOW TO GENTLY INCREASE CARDIO INTENSITY

Increasing aerobic intensity gradually is critical for boosting cardiovascular fitness and overall health while reducing the chance of damage. Here are some tips for effectively and safely increasing cardiac intensity for seniors:

1. Start with a baseline: Determine your current fitness level by engaging in a simple cardio activity, such as walking, at a comfortable rate. Take note of how long you can go without feeling exhausted. This will assist you in setting realistic short- and long-term goals.

2. Increase the duration gradually: Start by increasing the duration of your cardio activities by 5-10 minutes every week. For example, if you walk for 20 minutes today, attempt increasing it to 25 minutes the next week. Pay heed to your body's signals and stick with your current duration if you feel too tired or uncomfortable to continue until you're ready.

3. Increase frequency: Include an extra day of cardio activity in your weekly schedule. If you already do cardio three times a week, try adding a fourth session. Make sure you have rest days in between tough workouts to allow for healing. For example, alternate between exercise and rest/light activity days.

4. Adjust the intensity gradually: Change the pace of your cardio activities somewhat. Increase your walking pace from leisurely to vigorous. If you're cycling, bike a little faster. Make incremental changes over time to avoid overexertion.

5. Incorporate intervals: Incorporate interval training into your program by alternating between periods of high and low intensity. For example, walk rapidly for one minute then return to a comfortable speed for two minutes. As your fitness increases, gradually increase the duration of higher intensity intervals.

6. Use resistance: To boost the intensity of your workouts, incorporate resistance exercises. For example, if you're walking, take a route with gentle inclines or hills. If you're pedaling on a stationary bike, raise the resistance. This promotes strength development while also improving cardiovascular fitness.

7. Monitor heart rate: Keep track of your heart rate while exercising to verify that you are operating within a safe and effective zone. Use a heart rate monitor or take your pulse manually. As your fitness improves, progressively increase the goal heart rate zone.

8. Change Up Your Routine: Incorporate a variety of cardio activities to challenge your body in fresh ways. For example, switch between walking, cycling, swimming, and low-impact dance. This not only reduces boredom, but also works different muscle areas and improves overall fitness.

9. Stay Consistent: Consistency is essential for progressively increasing cardiac intensity. Stick to your fitness routine and make small, gradual modifications over time. Avoid making abrupt or extreme adjustments that could result in injury or fatigue.

10. Consult a professional: Consult your doctor or a fitness professional before making significant modifications to your cardio routine. They may offer tailored guidance based on your health and fitness objectives, ensuring that you increase intensity safely and successfully.

Following these guidelines allows seniors to gradually raise their cardio intensity, boosting cardiovascular health, endurance, and overall well-being while reducing the chance of injury.

MONITORING HEART RATE AND EXERCISE LEVELS

Monitoring heart rate and effort levels is critical for ensuring that cardiovascular exercise is safe and effective, particularly for the elderly. Keeping track of these data allows you to maintain a healthy exercise intensity range and avoid overexertion, which can lead to injury or other health issues.

Understanding Heart Rate

Resting heart rate (RHR) is the number of times your heart beats per minute (BPM) while at rest. Most adults have a resting heart rate of 60-100 beats per minute (BPM), however athletes may have a lower rate. The maximum heart rate (MHR) is the highest heart rate that an individual may achieve without causing serious difficulties. It is commonly calculated by subtracting your age from 220. For example, a 60-year-old would have an estimated MHR of 160 BPM (220 - 60 = 160). The target heart rate zone, which is 50-85% of your maximal heart rate, guarantees that you exercise at a safe and effective level.

Calculate Your Target Heart Rate Zone.

First, subtract your age from 220 to determine your maximum heart rate. Then, multiply your MHR by 0.5 and 0.85 to calculate the lower and upper bounds of your goal heart rate zone. For example, a 60-year-old's MHR is 160 BPM. The lower limit is 160 x 0.5 = 80 BPM, and the maximum limit is 160 x 0.85 = 136 BPM, resulting in the target heart rate zone 80-136 BPM.

Monitoring the Heart Rate

You can manually measure your heart rate by taking your pulse at your wrist or neck, noting the number of beats in 15 seconds, and multiplying by four to calculate your BPM. Wearable gadgets, such as fitness trackers or chest straps, can also be used as heart rate monitors, providing continuous and often more precise monitoring.

Understanding Exertion Levels

The rate of perceived exertion (RPE) is a subjective measure of how hard you believe you are working during exercise. The Borg Scale, which spans from 6 to 20, is widely used to assess this. A grade of 6 implies little exertion, whereas a rating of 20 indicates maximum intensity. For most cardio workouts, seniors should have an RPE of 12-14 (moderate to slightly challenging).

Combined Heart Rate and RPE

Using combined heart rate and RPE provides a complete picture of exercise intensity. If your heart rate is within the intended range but your RPE feels abnormally high, you may have overexerted. If your RPE feels too low, you may need to increase the effort to meet your fitness objectives.

Adjusting Exercise based on Monitoring

Regularly monitoring and modifying your workout intensity based on heart rate and RPE ensures that you exercise safely and successfully. If your heart rate frequently exceeds the target zone or your RPE is high, try lowering the intensity or taking additional rest breaks. If your heart rate is regularly lower than the goal zone and your RPE is low, gradually raise the intensity to test your cardiovascular system.

Seniors can safely improve their cardiovascular fitness by monitoring their heart rate and exercise levels, ensuring they remain below safe limits while gradually improving their health and endurance.

CONCLUSION

Maintaining physical fitness is critical for seniors, and a well-rounded home workout plan can greatly improve general health, mobility, and quality of life. The exercises and suggestions in this book are intended to be safe, effective, and pleasant for those over the age of 50, and will help you gain strength, flexibility, balance, and cardiovascular health.

You may lay the groundwork for a successful fitness journey by incorporating economical and space-saving training equipment, creating a safe exercise environment, and recognizing the value of thorough warm-ups. Regularly monitoring your heart rate and exertion levels ensures that you exercise safely, while gradually increasing intensity allows you to progress without risking damage.

Including a variety of exercises, such as stretching and balance, yoga, and cardio, addresses different elements of physical fitness. These activities not only improve your physical health, but they also help with mental clarity and emotional stability. Simple routines and changes ensure that each exercise is matched to your fitness level, allowing you to stay active and motivated.

Remember that consistency is crucial. Regularly practicing these exercises will result in significant improvements in your strength, endurance, and flexibility. Additionally, analyzing your success and tweaking routines as needed will keep you on track to meet your fitness goals.

Finally, a home workout routine designed for elders over 50 is an effective strategy for improving their long-term well-being. Follow the suggestions and activities in this book to live a healthier, more active lifestyle. Take this trip with confidence, knowing that every step is an investment in your health and pleasure. remain active, remain safe, and, most importantly, enjoy the journey of becoming a stronger, more vibrant version of yourself.